Karolinska Institute Nobel Conference Series

ETHICS IN MEDICINE
INDIVIDUAL INTEGRITY VERSUS DEMANDS OF SOCIETY

A Raven Press Rapid Publication

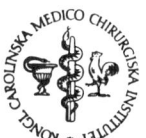

Karolinska Institute
Nobel Conference Series

Ethics in Medicine
Individual Integrity Versus Demands of Society

Editors

Peter Allebeck, M.D.
*Department of Medicine
Karolinska Institute at Huddinge
University Hospital
Stockholm, Sweden*

Bengt Jansson, M.D.
*Department of Psychiatry
Karolinska Institute at Huddinge
University Hospital
Stockholm, Sweden*

Congress Organizers

Shimon Glick, M.D.
*Ben-Gurion University of the Negev
Beersheva, Israel*

Bengt Jansson, M.D.
*Karolinska Institute
Stockholm, Sweden*

Elliot Leiter, M.D.
*Beth Israel Medical Center
New York, New York*

Raven Press ♦ New York

Raven Press Ltd., 1185 Avenue of the Americas, New York, New York 10036

© 1990 By Raven Press, Ltd. All rights reserved. This book is protected by copyright. No part of it may be reproduced, stored in a retrieval system, or transmitted, in any form or by any means, electronic, mechanical, photocopying, or recording, or otherwise, without the prior written permission of the publisher.

Made in the United States of America

Library of Congress Cataloging-in-Publication Data

Ethics in medicine.

(Karolinska Institute Nobel conference series)
"The Third International Congress on Ethics in
Medicine, held in Stockholm 1989"--Pref.
  Includes bibliographical references.
  1. Medical ethics--Congresses. I. Allebeck, Peter.
II. Jansson, Bengt. III. International Congress on
Ethics in Medicine (3rd : 1989 : Stockholm, Sweden)
IV. Series. [DNLM: 1. Delivery of Health Care--standards
--congresses. 2. Ethics, Medical--congresses. 3. Health
Policy--congresses. 4. Research--standards--congresses.
5. Social Values--congresses.   W 50 E8432 1989]
R724.E8234   1990   174'.2   90-8229
ISBN 0-88167-660-8

Papers or parts thereof have been used as camera-ready copy as submitted by the authors whenever possible; when retyped, they have been edited by the editorial staff only to the extent considered necessary for the assistance of an international readership. The views expressed and the general style adopted remain, however, the responsibility of the named authors. Great care has been taken to maintain the accuracy of the information contained in the volume. However, neither Raven Press nor the editors can be held responsible for errors or for any consequences arising from the use of information contained herein.

The use in this book of particular designations of countries or territories does not imply any judgment by the publisher or editors as to the legal status of such countries or territories, of their authorities or institutions, or of the delimitation of their boundaries.

Some of the names of products referred to in this book may be registered trademarks or proprietary names, although specific reference to this fact may not be made; however, the use of a name with designation is not to be construed as a representation by the publisher or editors that it is in the public domain. In addition, the mention of specific companies or of their products or proprietary names does not imply an endorsement or recommendation on the part of the publisher or editors.

Authors were themselves responsible for obtaining the necessary permission to reproduce copyright materials from other sources. With respect to the publisher's copyright, material appearing in this book prepared by individuals as part of their official duties as government employees is only covered by this copyright to the extent permitted by the appropriate national regulations.

9 8 7 6 5 4 3 2 1

Preface

Not long ago, medical ethics was a somewhat special discipline, mainly concerned with issues related to the beginning and end of life and with classic questions like abortion, euthanasia, and doctor–patient relationships. Research, debate, and policymaking were led by a limited number of strongly committed persons, who often had difficulty in promoting a broader debate and getting support for formalized research and training in medical ethics.

Over the last two decades, the interest in medical ethics has grown at a rapid rate along several lines: 1) ethical issues have become a central matter of concern in a large number of health-care activities, such as research, priority setting, patient rights, and high-technology medicine; 2) the interdisciplinary character of medical ethics has grown to include many different categories of health-care workers, philosophers, theologians, lawyers, policymakers, and many other professional groups; (3) the focus of the debate is not only doctors and patients in a hospital setting, but more and more interactions between the general public (prospective patients, relatives, research subjects, patients on a waiting list) and the health-care system and those who plan and organize health-care services (politicians and administrators).

It was against this background that the first world congress on ethics in medicine was held in Israel in 1985. The collaboration of three institutions—the Beth Israel Medical Center, New York, New York, U.S.A., the Ben-Gurion University of the Negev, Beersheva, Israel, and the Karolinska Institute, Stockholm, Sweden—ensured the continuation of a series of international congresses on ethics in medicine: in New York in 1987 and in Stockholm in 1989. Efforts are being made to incorporate other institutions in other countries to make this series a truly international forum for deliberations on ethics in medicine.

This book is divided into five sections: integrity and autonomy, clinical freedom, priorities in medical health care, ethical problems in epidemiological research, and ethical aspects on HIV.

Integrity and autonomy is a classic theme in medical ethics that has become even more important with the development of high-technology medicine, the HIV problem, and new forms of medical research. Furthermore, setting priorities has become a crucial issue in health-care planning all over the world. The problems in setting priorities and the different solutions that have been put forward in bone marrow transplantation, cardiology, and care for the elderly are delineated.

The term "clinical freedom" is often heard but rarely analyzed in terms of what really are the limits to clinical freedom for physicians and health-care workers. Rights and limitations for physicians *and* patients are discussed in this section.

The development of new methods in epidemiological research has prompted a debate on ethical aspects and the need for ethical guidelines for researchers. Key issues of this debate are presented, as well as possibilities and problems in formulating ethical guidelines for this type of research.

Finally, the various problems related to HIV infection actualize most ethical issues encountered in medicine: integrity, autonomy, research ethics, society's demands, etc. Examples are given from the clinical setting, from the research perspective, and from the political and administrative point of view.

This book will be of interest to many professional groups as well as patient groups and other laymen who have taken an interest in the broad field of medical ethics. Physicians and other health-care workers, lawyers, theologians, health-care administrators, and politicians are faced almost daily with problems related to medical ethics. This volume will enable the reader to expand his or her knowledge of this field.

The Editors

Acknowledgments

This book is based on plenary lectures delivered at the Third International Congress on Ethics in Medicine, held in Stockholm, Sweden, in 1989.

We thank our colleagues, Professor Shimon Glick at the Ben-Gurion University of the Negev, Beersheva, Israel, and Dr. Elliot Leiter at the Beth Israel Medical Center, New York, New York, U.S.A., for the collaboration in the preparation of the congress. We are indebted to The Nobel Assembly at the Karolinska Institute, the Kjell and Märta Beijer Foundation, The Swedish Society of Medicine, and the Commission for Social Research (DSF) for financial support. We also thank Pia Inoue for skillful typing and secretarial assistance in the preparation of this volume.

Contents

Integrity and Autonomy

1 Introduction
L. Jacobsson

3 The Relationship of Autonomy and Integrity in Medical Ethics
E. D. Pellegrino

23 The Roots of Medical Ethics in a Shared Morality
K. E. Tranöy

33 Integrity and Autonomy from an Anthropological Point of View
L. Sachs

47 The Ideas of Integrity and Autonomy: Discussion
E. Bischofberger

Priorities in Medical Health Care

53 Introduction
G. Gahrton

55 Setting Limits in Health Care
D. Callahan

65 Priorities for Treatment with Highly Specialized Technology—Bone Marrow Transplantation
G. Gahrton

69 Priorities for Advanced Technology in the Diagnosis and Treatment of Patients with Heart Disorders
O. Edhag

77 Rationing and Priority Setting: Discussion
S. Glick

Clinical Freedom

89 Clinical Freedom: Where are the Limits to the Freedom of Doctors?
R. Hoffenberg

103 Clinical Freedom: Patients' and Physicians' Autonomy Versus the Demands of Society
P. Riis

115 On Doctors and Patients
A. Carmi

Ethical Problems in Epidemiological Research

123 Introduction
C.-G. Westrin

125 An Ethical Framework for Epidemiology
J. M. Last

137 Ethical Guidelines and Codes—Can They be Universally Applicable in a Multi-Cultural World?
E. Keyserlingk

151 Ethical Aspects on Epidemiological Research
P. Allebeck

159 Ethical and Legal Problems in Researcher's Access to Data Stores
J. Benbassat and M. Levy

167 Ethical Problems in Epidemiological Research: Discussion
G. Hermerén

Ethical Aspects on HIV

179 Introduction
B. Jansson

181 HIV Infection and Parenteral Drug Abuse: Ethical Issues in Diagnosis, Treatment, Research, and the Maintenance of Confidentiality
M. J. Kreek

189 Medical Versus Political Aspects of Creating a Policy Against a Severe Disaster
B. Westerholm

199 Ethical Issues in Clinical Practice
O. Berglund

203 Public Health Measures with HIV Infection: A Model for Identification and Analysis of Ethical Conflicts
T. Nilstun

215 Subject Index

Contributors

Peter Allebeck
Section for Community Medicine
Karolinska Institute at Huddinge
  University Hospital
S-141 86 Stockholm, Sweden

Jochanan Benbassat
Department of Medicine
Hadassah University
Hospital al Ein Kerem
Jerusalem 91240, Israel

Ove Berglund
Department of Infectious Diseases
Karolinska Institute at Roslagstull
  Hospital
S-114 89 Stockholm, Sweden

Erwin Bischofberger
National Medical Ethics Council
Tidskr Signum St. Johannesg 22 B
S-752 35 Uppsala, Sweden

Daniel Callahan
Hastings Center
255 Elm Road
Briarcliff Manor, New York 10510

Amnon Carmi
World Association of Medical Law
University of Haifa
Mount Carmel
Haifa 31999, Israel

Olof Edhag
Department of Medicine
Karolinska Institute at Huddinge
  University Hospital
S-141 86 Stockholm, Sweden

Gösta Gahrton
Department of Medicine
Karolinska Institute at Huddinge
  University Hospital
S-141 86 Stockholm, Sweden

Shimon Glick
Faculty of Health Sciences
Ben-Gurion University of the Negev
P.O. Box 653
Beersheva, Israel

Göran Hermerén
Department of Philosophy
University of Lund
S-223 50 Lund, Sweden

Sir Raymond Hoffenberg
Royal College of Physicians
11 St. Andrews Place
Regent Park
London NW1 4LE, United Kingdom

Lars Jacobsson
Department of Psychiatry
University of Umeå
S-901 85 Umeå, Sweden

Bengt Jansson
Department of Psychiatry
Karolinska Institute at Huddinge
  University Hospital
S-141 86 Stockholm, Sweden

Edward Keyserlingk
The McGill Centre for Medicine,
  Ethics and Law
1110 Pain Avenue West
Montreal, Quebec, Canada H3A 1A3

Mary Jeanne Kreek
Rockefeller University
1230 York Avenue
New York, New York 10021-6399

John M. Last
Department of Epidemiology and
  Community Medicine
Faculty of Health Sciences
University of Ottawa
451 Smyth
Ottawa, Ontario, Canada K12 8M5

Micha Levy
Department of Medicine
Hadassah University
Hospital al Ein Kerem
Jerusalem 91240, Israel

Tore Nilstun
Department of Philosophy
University of Lund
S-223 50 Lund, Sweden

Edmund D. Pellegrino
Center for Advanced Study of Ethics and
John Carroll Professor of Medicine and
  Medical Humanities
Georgetown University
Washington, DC 20057

Povl Riis
Department of Internal Medicine
University of Copenhagen
Herlev Hospital
DK-2730 Herlev, Denmark

Lisbeth Sachs
Department of International Health Care
  Research
Karolinska Institute
S-104 01 Stockholm, Sweden

Knut Erik Tranöy
Department of General Medicine
University of Oslo
NO2264 Oslo 2, Norway

Barbro Westerholm
Department of Pharmacology
Apoteksbelaget AB
Member of Parliament
S-105 14 Stockholm, Sweden

Claes-Göran Westrin
Department of Social Medicine
University of Uppsala
S-751 85 Uppsala, Sweden

Karolinska Institute Nobel Conference Series

Ethics in Medicine: Individual Integrity Versus Demands of Society
Peter Allebeck and Bengt Jansson, Editors; 240 pp., 1990

Growth Factors: From Genes to Clinical Application
Vicki R. Sara, Kerstin Hall, and Hans Löw, Editors; 288 pp., 1990

Neuropeptide Y
Viktor Mutt, Kjell Fuxe, Tomas Hökfelt, and Jan M. Lundberg, Editors; 376 pp., 1989

Pathogenesis of Non-Insulin Dependent Diabetes Mellitus
Valdemar Grill and Suad Efendić, Editors; 336 pp., 1988

Neurobiology of the Control of Breathing
Curt von Euler and Hugo Lagercrantz, Editors; 352 pp., 1987

Thioredoxin and Glutaredoxin Systems: Structure and Function
Arne Holmgren, Carl-Ivar Brändén, Hans Jörnvall, and Britt-Marie Sjoberg, Editors; 430 pp., 1986

Karolinska Institute Nobel Conference Series

ETHICS IN MEDICINE
INDIVIDUAL INTEGRITY VERSUS DEMANDS OF SOCIETY

Ethics in Medicine, edited by
Peter Allebeck and Bengt Jansson.
Raven Press, New York © 1990.

INTEGRITY AND AUTONOMY

INTRODUCTION

Lars Jacobsson

The concept of integrity has become very crucial in the debate on medical ethics for many reasons. The integrity of the donor's body is the most important question in the transplantation issue. The prevention and treatment of HIV-infection is strongly dependent on the possibilities to find a solution to the dilemma of caring for the integrity and autonomy of the HIV-infected individual, and the legitimate demands of protection and security from the rest of the population. Integrity is also a very central issue in research. The use of data registers for example, is very much a matter of how to respect the individual and his integrity and autonomy in the concern for the health of the general population. Another example is the possibilities of using modern gene-technique to manipulate the genetics of man.

This section on "integrity and autonomy" will deal with the issue of integrity and autonomy from a theoretical point of view.

Professor Edmund Pellegrino of the Kennedy

Institute of Ethics, Georgetown University, Washington, USA, will introduce the subject based on his background as an internist.

Professor Knut Erik Tranöy, the Institution of General Medicine, University of Oslo, Norway, who is originally a philosopher, but for the last years has been professor of medical ethics in Oslo, will discuss integrity and autonomy from the philosophical point of view, departing from the idea that bioethics/medical ethics is not different from "ordinary" general ethics.

In a third paper Associated Professor Lisbeth Sachs at the Karolinska Institute in Stockholm, will give a social antropologist's view on integrity and identity. Integrity is very much linked to identity and identity is very much a matter of social roles and cultural factors.

These three introductory papers will be commented on by dr Erwin Bischofberger. He is a jesuit father and lecturer in medical ethics at the Karolinska Institute in Stockholm and at the university of Uppsala, with a theological background.

THE RELATIONSHIP OF AUTONOMY AND INTEGRITY IN MEDICAL ETHICS

Edmund D. Pellegrino

> Integrity without knowledge is weak and useless, and knowledge without integrity is dangerous and dreadful.
> Samuel Johnson, Rasselas, 1759.

Introduction

In the last twenty-five years autonomy has superceded beneficence as the first principle of medical ethics. This is the most radical reorientation in the long history of the Hippocratic tradition. As a result, the physician-patient relationship has become more honest, open, and respectful of the dignity of patients.

This shift in the locus of decision-making is a response to the coalescence of socio-political, legal, and ethical forces that make it well nigh irreversible. The central ethical question today is not whether patient autonomy will remain a predominant principle. Rather, the issue is a critical assessment of its full impact on the relationships between physicians and patients. Does the principle of autonomy as now construed encompass the full meaning of respect for the dignity of persons? May the tendency to absolutize autonomy defeat some of the purposes for which it has been so vigorously propounded? Is there a deeper source for the principle of autonomy that more fully encompasses the special nuances required in authentic respect for persons?

In this essay I shall argue: 1) that autonomy as now construed has certain moral and practical limitations; 2) that these limitations can be ameliorated by linking autonomy to the principle of respect for the integrity of persons; and 3) that this move encompasses a more fundamental and richer safeguard for the dignity of both patient and physician than current interpretations of the principle of autonomy.

I shall attempt to advance these propositions by examining the following: 1) the origins and nature of the concept and principle of autonomy and its expression in today's paradigm for ethical decision-making; 2) the concept and principle of integrity, its relationships to autonomy, and the distinctions between them; and 3) the relationship of the principles of autonomy and the integrity of persons to the virtue of integrity.

1. Autonomy - origins and nature, as concept and principle

Autonomy, despite its universal usage in medical ethics, is too often simplistically interpreted, as Faden and Beauchamp have so cogently pointed out (1). For example, they make a sharp and valid distiction between the autonomous person and the autonomous action, preferring in their treatment of informed consent to emphasize the autonomous act, rather than the autonomous person. While agreeing with their distinction, this essay will place more emphasis on the autonomous person and on the relationship of that concept to the concept of the integrity of persons which underlies it.

Autonomy, in keeping with its Greek etymology, literally means self-rule. In today's parlance, autonomy has variously been interpreted as a moral and legal claim, a right, duty, concept or principle. I shall take it, for purposes of this essay, as a capacity for self-rule, a quality inherent in rational beings that enables them to make reasoned choices and actions based on a personal assessment of future possibilities evaluated in terms of their own value systems. On this view, autonomy is a capacity that flows from the fact that humans can think and feel and make judgements about what they seem to be good.

The universal existence of this capacity in rational beings does not guarantee that it can, or will function fully or at all. There are internal and external constraints which can impede autonomous decisions and actions. Internal constraints include such things as brain damage or dysfunction induced by disordered metabolic states, drugs or injury, or lack of mental competence related to infancy and childhood, mental retardation or psychoses, obsessive-compulsive neuroses, etc. In these instances the physiological substratum requisite to the exercise of the capacity for autonomy is impaired - sometimes reversibly, sometimes not.

Autonomy may be unimpaired internally yet be prevented from operation by external events like coercion, physical and emotional deception, or deprivation of essential information. In these cases the person has the capacity for self-rule but that capacity cannot be realized in an autonomous action, i.e. an action which gives evidence of "autonomous authorization" (2). An autonomous act satisfies the criteria for informed consent. It is a decision and act free from internal or external constraints, informed as fully as the situation requires, and consistent with the person's evaluation, at the moment of choice, of the person's own value system.

The existence of the capacity for self-rule is so deeply embedded in what it means to be a human being that it constitutes a moral claim, a claim which generates a duty of respect in other persons. This claim is expressed as the priniple of autonomy: ie., so act in relationships with others that their capacity for autonomy (and thus their moral claim) can be exercised as fully as circumstances will permit.

1.A <u>Social and political sources</u>

The recent shift in the locus of the decision from physician to patient, while seemingly abrupt, had been developing in the Western world since the birth, in the eighteenth century, of the modern idea of a participatory democracy. This article is not the place to review that history. We need only enumerate the socio-political forces that coalesced in the mid-sixties to place autonomy in the forefront of medical ethics legally and philosophically: the Nuremberg trials; the worldwide spread of participatory democracy; mistrust of authority in general and technical expertise in particular; the expansion of public education; the civil rights movement; the intrusions of law, economics, and commerce into medical decisions; and the challenges of bio-technology that had to be faced in a progressively pluralistic society that could muster little moral consensus.

These forces converged to engender mistrust of the physician's traditional paternalism and a demand for self-determination and informed consent in medical relationships. "Autonomy" has become the watchword that symbolizes the moral and legal claim of patients to make their own decisions without constraint or coercion, however beneficent the physician's intentions might be. The socio-political claim to autonomous decision and action was re-entered by the legal concept of privacy and by the philosophic principle of autonomy.

1.B The legal basis for individual autonomy

Though still debated among legal scholars the legal basis for the claim to autonomy is usually grounded in the right to privacy (3). Such a right is not specifically stated in the American Constitution, but has been derived, in a series of Supreme Court decisions, as a "penumbra" of several amendments of the Bill of Rights (4). This right to privacy has, in practical terms, been applied to the right of personal decision regarding the education of children, choice of a marriage partner, religious preference, access to contraceptive devices and termination of pregnancy (5). This same right has been explicitly invoked to protect a patient's right to refuse medical treatments (6).

In the last two decades, the legal right to self-determination has been progressively extended from the patient to his or her surrogate, from mechanical respirators to food and fluid, from terminal to non-terminal patients, and from the patient himself to his or her living will (7). The legal right to self-determination and privacy has acted as a powerful restraint on the traditional benevolent paternalism of the physician. It has also acted as an impetus for the doctrine of informed consent.

1.C The philosophic roots

The principle of autonomy has several sources in moral philosophy. One is Locke's "Second Treatise on Government", which held man in the state of nature to be free and equal so that none might have sovereignity over another except through a social contract freely entered into (8). Locke's arguments gave rise to the notion of "negative rights" - rights of a person not to be interfered with by others. These negative rights have come to be the foundation of liberal democracy for many people (9).

A second, powerful and influential philosophical moral claim to autonomy is propounded in Kant's "Groundwork for the Metaphysics of Morals" (10). Here Kant argues that freedom is essential to all morality, that it is identical with autonomy, and that autonomy is "the ground of the dignity of human nature and of every rational nature" (11). Kant unites the idea of a rational being with dignity this way: "... a rational being himself must be the ground for all maxims of action never merely as a means, but as a sypreme condition restricting the use of every means, that is, always also as an end" (12). "And the dignity of man consists precisely in his capacity to make universal law, although only on condition of being himself subject to the law he makes" (13).

A third source for a moral claim to autonomy is John S. Mill's essay "On Liberty" (14). Mill asserts that the only restraint on liberty is harm to others, not harm to self. This latter notion, joined with the Lockean idea of negative rights, is the major connecting link between the philosophical notion of autonomy and the legal notion of privacy. This link is most influential with the courts in America. It is the principle generally used to resolve conflicts about who should make the final decision in accepting or rejecting medical treatment. It is the dominant concept as well in the report of the President's Commission on the withholding and withrawing life sustaining treatment (15).

This conjunction of the legal concept of privacy and the moral concept of autonomy has resulted in a widely accepted medical decision-making paradigm: Competent patients have the moral and legal right to make their own decisions, and these decisions take precedence over those of the doctor or the family. When patients are no longer competent (or have never been competent, e.g. infants, the retarded), their rights of decision are transferred to a valid surrogate or to some anticipatory statement by the patient (e.g. a living will, medical directive or durable power of attorney) or in the absence of these to a legally appointed guardian. Some have so absolutized the principle of autonomy and the right of privacy that they would place no limits on its exercise. Others accept varying degrees of limitation on autonomy. We shall return to these exceptions later when we examine the links between autonomy and integrity.

The most concrete actualization of the principles of privacy and autonomy lies in the doctrine of informed consent which has become the central requirement of morally valid medical decision-making. For consent to fulfill the claims of human persons to self-governance, it must be based on sufficient information to make a reasoned choice and must be free of coercion or deception. The procedures surrounding informed consent are designed to facilitate the capacity of rational beings to make judgements of what they consider best rather than what the physician or any other person might consider best for them.

1.D <u>Deficiencies of autonomy as a moral guide</u>

There can be no question of the importance of the socio-political, legal, and moral emphasis on autonomy in protecting the patient's right of self-determination. But there are certain limitations to the concept of autonomy itself that may impede the fullest expressions of the respect for persons which autonomy is supposed to enhance.

For one thing, autonomy has come to have a strong legalistic quality centering all too often on invasion of privacy, assault, battery, and tort law in general. Such conceptions tend to moral minimalism, i.e., to fulfillment only of what is specifically prescribed. Documentary evidence and protection against lawsuit become almost obsessive concerns, rather than the moral quality of the consent process. This focus fosters the all-too-

-frequent notion of the physician-patient relationship as a contract rather than a fiduciary relationship or a covenant. The fiction is encouraged that a contract is possible in a relationship in which one party is ill, vulnerable, and exploitable and the other holds the needed knowledge and power. On the contractural view, the procedures for making a valid informed consent, important as they are, come to take the place of the substantive moral issue itself.

A strong emphasis on self-determination also minimizes the physician's obligations of beneficence and effacement of self-interest. Some even see beneficence as antipathetic to autonomy - a false dichotomy I shall treat a little further on in this essay. Autonomy, when viewed as a legal right or even as a moral claim, can severely circumscribe the range of discretionary decisions - those unanticipated choices the clinical situation may force on the physician. Ordinarily the physician would feel free to act in the patient's best interests as he himself perceives them. For example, the proposed "medical directive," which consists of six pages of detailed instruction on how the physician should manage life-sustaining and other treatments, could easily lead to a paralysis of decision-making injurious to the patient (16). When patients are unable to spell out everything in advance, the physician may spend more time trying to figure out what the patient wishes than deciding what is in the patient's interests.

Finally, the prevailing emphasis on autonomy generates a cult of moral privatism, atomism, and individualism that is insensitive to the fact that humans are member of a moral community. When autonomy is absolutized, each person is a moral atom who asserts his or her rights independently and even against the claims of the social entity to which he/she belongs. Conflicts between the rights of a community and of its individual members raise serious questions of economic and social justice that demand a better balance between autonomy and the common good than now obtains.

Many of the moral shortcomings of the concept and principle of autonomy are ameliorated if we look to the more fundamental concept of integrity of persons of which autonomy is a partial, but not a full, expression.

2. Integrity of persons and persons of integrity

Etymologically, integrity is from the Latin "integer", and it means wholeness, completeness, or unimpaired unity. It is a more complex notion than autonomy. Integrity encompasses autonomy, because loss of autonomy impairs acting as an intact and whole human being. But autonomy is not synonymous with integrity of the person since integrity includes physiological, psychological, and spiritual wholeness. Autonomy is a capacity of the whole person, but not the whole of a person's capacities. As Karol Wojtyla puts it, "integration is an essential condition for the transcendence of the person in the whole of the psychosomatic compexity of the human subject" (17). Gabriel Marcel puts it this way: "I want to run my own life" is "the radical formula of autonomy". Autonomy belongs to the order of <u>having</u>, to the things we possess, while true freedom belongs to the order of <u>being</u>, to what we <u>are</u>. On this view freedom may paradoxically even include non-freedom (18).

Integrity has two senses of significance for medical ethics. One sense refers to the integrity of the person, of the patient, and of the physician; the other refers to being a person of integrity. In the first sense, integrity is a moral claim which belongs to every human simply by virtue of being human. In the second sense, integrity is a virtue, a moral habitus acquired by constant practice in our relation with others. Integrity belongs to all persons as humans, but not all are persons of integrity. Each sense of integrity has important ethical implications in medical ethics.

2.A <u>Integrity of the person</u>

By the integrity of the person we mean the right ordering of the parts to the whole, the balance and harmony between the various dimensions of human existence necessary for the well functioning of the whole human organism. The integrity of a person is expressed in a balanced relationship between the bodily, psycho-social, and intellectual elements of his or her life. No one element is out of proportion to the others. Each takes the lead when the good of the whole requires it. Each yields to the other in the interest of the whole. Integrity in this sense is synonymous with health. Disease amounts to disintegration, a rupture of the unity of the person

(19). This rupture may occur in one or more of three spheres, each with its own ethical implications: the corporeal, the psychological, and the axiological.

Bodily integrity implies a well-functioning organism physiologically, a body which can serve the aims and purposes of the person efficiently and effectively with a minimum of discomfort or disability. With physical illness, corporeal unity is shattered. The body (or one of its organs) becomes the focus of attention and loses some or all of its capacity for work, play, or human relationships. There may even be loss of an organ or a function. The functional integrity of the whole organism is disrupted by a sick organ, organ system, or metabolic mechanism.

Illness may also assault the psychological integrity of the person in two ways. In one way, emotional illness is a form of dis-integration in which anxieties, obsessions, compulsions, illusions, and other psychopathological disorders assume control of existence. The resulting distortions of the balance and unity of the person interfere with his/her well-functioning as much as the rupture of corporeal unity.

Another form of psychological integrity is the unity of the self in its relationship to the body. When illness afflicts a part of the body, we feel alienated from that part, we stand in some senses away from the offending body, we sometimes reject it and resent it as an enemy. The image we have fashioned of our self-identity in relationship to our bodily integrity is threatened. We all live with a unique balance we have struck over the years between our hopes and aspirations and the limitations imposed by our physiological, psychological, or physical shortcomings. Serious illness forces a confrontation with the impact of disability, pain, and death on that image. It confronts us with the possibility of a substantially altered self-image or even non-existence. A new image, new points of balance, and a new definition of what constitutes health must be established if we are to become "whole" again.

Another facet of the integrity of persons is axiological integrity, i.e., the intactness of the values we cherish and espouse. Each of us is in a real sense defined by the particular configuration of values we have chosen as our own. In illness these values may be in conflict with those of the physician, our families, or society. Our conception of healing reflects our personal assessment of what constitutes well functioning. This is as much a value determined conception as it is physical or psychological. In order for us to be cured or treated, our most cherished values must also become the subject of the physician's scrutiny and possible manipulation. Our values thus are at risk of challenge or damage in the medical transaction.

The potential for the tri-partite dis-integration of the person, which is part of being ill, creates obligations for the physician who is bound by covenant to heal and help. Healing means to make whole again, that is, to re-establish the wholeness that constitutes a healthy existence. To be faithful to this covenant the physician is obliged to remedy the dis-integration of the person inflicted by disease. On this view, restoration of the integrity of the person is the moral basis of the physician-patient relationship. That is why any morally authentic doctor - patient relationship must by definition be "wholistic".

In illness the vulnerability of the patient's body, psyche, and values generates the obligation to enhance and restore the patient's autonomous capacity for decision-making. Autonomy is thus grounded ultimately in the integrity of the person. To usurp the patient's human capacity for self-governance is to violate that integrity. To ignore, override, repudiate or ridicule the patient's values is to assault the patient's very humanity. This affront aggravates the dis-integration of the person already there as a result of illness. Nothing could be further from a morally defensible healing relationship.

Paradoxically, to repair the dis-integration produced by disease the integrity of the person must to some degree be violated. The physician lays hands on the patient, pers into every orifice, inquires into the details of the patient's social relationships and psychological responses. This is a licit invasion of integrity to which the patient gives assent. But consent cannot obviate the exposure of integrity to serious risk attendant on medical treatment. This is another source of moral obligation which binds the physician to exercise the right to necessary invasions of integrity with the utmost care and sensitivity.

2.B Limitations of the patient's claim to autonomy

However fundamental, the patient's moral claim to respect for his integrity and autonomy is not absolute. There are several limitations that arise when the patient's moral claim conflicts with the equivalent claims to integrity made by other persons.

One such limitation is the claim of the physician, as a person, to his own autonomy. The patient cannot violate the physician's integrity as a person. If the physician is morally opposed to abortion, euthanasia, withdrawal or withholding of food or fluid, or artificial insemination, for example, he cannot be expected to comply with the patient's autonomy and suppress the integrity of his own person. This will become an increasingly important matter as morally debatable procedures such as voluntary and involuntary euthanasia become legalized or, eventually perhaps, benefits of health insurance. Both physician and patient are obliged to respect the integrity of each other's person; neither may impose his/her values on the other. Respectful withdrawal from the relationship may be necessary for the physician or the patient to avoid cooperation in acts which might compromise personal moral integrity.

Another limitation on a patient's autonomous decision occurs when action might produce a serious, definable, and direct harm to another person. An example here is the patient who is HIV seropositive and refuses to have that fact revealed to his or her spouse or sexual partner. In this instance the physician cannot withdraw, but he/she has the obligation in justice to tell the person at risk, after first offering the patient the opportunity to reveal the fact himself/herself. The same limitation applies to the patient who wishes to conceal some health problem which might compromise his/her capacity to fulfill a position of trust - e.g., a pilot, surgeoin, or cleric.

The autonomous decision of a valid surrogate must also be resisted if there is clear evidence of a conflict of interest, which might lead to the over- or under-treatment of an infant or incompetent adult. The physicina's primary obligation is the preservation of the integrity of the person of his patient.

Under cirumstances like these, the physician cannot withdraw but must take the measures available in a democratic society to protect the patient's interests. This protection may mean reference to an ethics committee, appointment of a legal guardian, or court intervention to limit the autonomy of the surrogates in emergencies, when the outcome is in doubt and when, in the absence of a specific instruction, the physician must act in the patient's best medical interests at least until the patient's wishes are clear.

Finally, the patient may on the moral strength of his/her own moral claim to autonomy yield up his/her claim to autonomy. Sometimes the physician has made a sincere effort to involve the competent patient yet the patient does not wish to participate as fully as other might. The patient might then ask that the physician should decide what is "best". Under such conditions, and only these, the physician has a moral mandate to decide for the patient - that is, to act in the patient's place and in the patient's interests. Not to do so is a form of moral abandonment. But the physician must never assume this mandate nor accept it too eagerly or lightly.

Carried to extremes the morally justifiable claim to autonomy could erode the communality of human existence. Autonomy absolutized leads to moral atomism, privatism, and anarchy. Humans are social animals. They cannot be fulfilled except in social relationships, as Aristotle so wisely pointed out (20). The community within which the patient resides has moral claims as well. This communitarian dimension of biomedical ethics is in danger of compromise if the current drive for autonomy is not modulated and balanced against the moral claims of other persons and the community.

The community, too, has a claim to integrity, i.e., to the same kind of wholeness, completeness, and intactness to which the individual lays claim. The fabric of a society can be torn, and the existence of society itself threatened, if individuals retreat into private morality independent of the community. We are in some danger of this when individuals or groups with special interests irresponsibly use resources common to all. Economically, the entrepreneur threatens the integrity of society when he despoils the environment. To a certain degree so do physicians, patients, or families who demand and use scarce medical resources when treatment is futile or the benefits disproportionate to the costs.

Patients, therefore, owe a debt to the community for the lifelong benefits they derive from being members of human communities. They should feel some duty to limit their demands for expensive or marginally beneficial treatments and technologies that impose financial burdens on society and their families. Out of a sense of social justice, voluntary limitations should be placed on life-support measures that are futile or that merely prolong the act of dying.

Finally, if we look at autonomy as a derivative of the integrity of the person and not as an isolated ethical principle, the presumed conflict between autonomy and beneficence should disappear. Paternalism could not be equated with beneficence, as some authors propose (21). Paternalism involves the physician's usurpation of the patient's moral claim as a human being to decide what is in his or her own best interests. This action violates the integrity of the person and could under no circumstances be a beneficent act. Rather, to be beneficent, respect for the patient's values and choices is essential. As Thomasma and I have pointed out elsewhere, the physician holds beneficence in trust (22), a point I will enlarge upon a little later.

2.C <u>Autonomy and integrity contrasted</u>

We may summarize the differences between autonomy and integrity in the following way: Autonomy is a capacity inherent in being a rational person. It is something we have or possess. If we have never developed our capacity for rational judgement, we do not have autonomy, and we can lose our autonomy when we lose this rational capacity. We can have degrees of autonomy depending on the interactions of internal and external impediments to the operation of our capacity for self-determined choices and actions. Under these circumstances our right to autonomy can be transferred to the decisions of a morally valid proxy or to a document like a living will, a durable power of attorney or medical directive. To transfer our autonomy is to violate an important part of our humanity, but it does not deprive us of our status as human persons.

Integrity, on the other hand, is a matter of being. It is an attribute possessed by all human beings competent or not, adult or infant, conscious or not. It does not admit of degrees nor can it be lost. Integrity is not something we have. It is part of our being as humans. It cannot be transferred to someone else. To violate our integrity is to violate our whole being as humans.

2.D Integrity of the decision

The principle of respect for the integrity can and does ameliorate some of the deficiencies of the principle of autonomy. For one thing respect for integrity is inconsistent with the minimalistic view of some physicians - namely, that autonomy is reducible to terms of a right to refuse treatment. In order truly to respect the integrity of the person, we must strive to give integrity to his/her decison as well, a wholeness that places that decision within the history and the background of the patient's life. A particular decision can never stand isolated from the whole narrative of the patient's life, the drama he or she has lived and is living, and the way he or she perceives self, family, and community in relation to the decision in question. Why, how, and what of the doctor's recommendations that the patient accepts or refuses must enter into the final choice if that choice is to have integrity in itself and be the act or decision of a whole or complete person.

Respect for integrity of persons also moves the patient's decision from the level of simple assent or dissent to the level of consent - i.e., the mutual and consensual arrival at a decision by doctor and patient acting together. On this view, respect for the integrity of persons requires a positive effort to get not just a decision that is autonomous by external criteria but one that represents the ground of knowing and feeling that exists between doctor and patient. It is not a case of patient assenting or dissenting as an isolated entity but doctor and patient consenting, that is, acting together, with each respecting the integrity of the other's person.

3. The person of integrity

The law of privacy, the principle of autonomy, and respect for the integrity of persons are necessary but not sufficient fully to preserve the integrity of the sick person in the medical transaction. What is indispensable is the person of integrity, the person of moral wholeness, who can be trusted to respect the nuances and subtleties of the moral claim to autonomy. The physician, therefore, must be a person who exhibits the virtue of integrity, a person who not only accepts respect for the autonomy of others as a principle or concept but also can be trusted to interpret its application in the most morally sensitive way.

The ultimate safeguard of the integrity of the patient's person is the fidelity of the physician to the trust inherent in the healing relationship. It is the physician who interprets and applies the principle of autonomy. Much depends upon how the physician presents the facts, which facts he/she selects and emphasizes, how much and how little he/she reveals, how he/she weighs risks and benefits, how he/she respects or exploits the fears and anxieties unique to his/her patient: in sum, how he/she uses his/her "Aesculaean power". Every patient, the most educated and the most independent, is potentially a victim or a beneficiary of that power. The resultant responsibility is heavy on the physician to be sensitive to the dependent, vulnerable, and frightened state of the patient and not to exploit that state even if the physician deems it is in the patient's best interests.

Clearly, no contract, law, or abstract ethical principle can eradicate the need for trust, just as trust cannot be eradicated from any other human relationship. The present emphasis on autonomy has served to reduce the grosser violations of the integrity of persons. But the physician's character remains the ultimate safeguard of the patient's autonomous wishes.

The physician is the pathway through which decicions, actions, and policies relating to the patient must pass. He or she is in a position to enhance and protect the patient's capacity for self-determination. This sensitive position does not give the physician privileges but only a heightened responsibility to be a steward of the moral quality of the healing relationship and the integrity of the person of the patient. The physician must never forget that he/she is automatically a moral accomplice in any policy, act, or decision that endangers the patient's integrity and autonomy. The fiduciary relationship is never entirely eradicable from the medical relationship. The physician must therefore be a person of integrity and cultivate the virtue of fidelity to trust. In fact, fidelity is perhaps the most fundamental of the virtues of the physician - as essential as beneficence and effacement of self-interest (23).

The relationships between autonomy, integrity, and trust which I have outlined for the medical relationship are of course not unique. But the nature of illness, what it portends physically and emotionally, and the invasions of the integrity of persons which are entailed in being healed - taken together - form a constellation of obligations rarely encountered in other kinds of human activity. Medical ethics is, to be sure, a part of general moral philosophy but an exquisitely sensitive part, given the phenomenology of being sick, being healed, and offering to heal.

For these reasons, a formula for morally defensible decision-making appears to be this: The decision should nor be made by the physician in place of the patient, nor by the patient in isolation from the physician or the community. Phenomenologically these elements of a medical decision are inseparable from each other. The morally optimal condition is one in which the decision arises between doctor and patient. For his or her part the physician should make the decision for, and with, the patient - the "for" signifying not "in place of", but "in the interests of" the patient. This formulation preserves the legal right to privacy, the moral claim to autonomy, and the deeper moral claim to the integrity of persons.

<u>Summary</u>

The emergence of autonomy as a socio-political, legal, and moral consept has profoundly influenced medical ethics. It has shifted the center of decision-making from the physician to the patient and re-oriented the whole physician-patient relationship in a revolutionary way. This has, on the whole, been salubrious. It has made the medical relationship more open, more honest, and more respectful of the dignity of the person of the patient. All in all, the ascendance of autonomy has protected patients against the grosser violations of autonomy and integrity so generally accepted as ethically permissible in the past. While much is still to be accomplished, the emergence of autonomy is an increasingly effective safeguard of the patient's dignity as a person.

But autonomy, while necessary as a principle of medical ethics, is insufficient to guarantee the nuances, the subtleties, and the full meanings of respect for persons in medical transactions. As a foundation for medical relationships, the concept of integrity is richer, more fundamental, and more closely tied to what it is to be a whole human person - corporeally, psychologically, and axiologically. The moral implications of integrity of persons are more demanding albeit more difficult to capture in legal language or in the procedures of informed consent. Yet for the reasons outlined in this paper, we should deepen our grasp of the notion of integrity of persons and come to the realization that autonomy depends upon preserving the integrity of persons and that both integrity of persons and autonomy depend on the physician being a person of integrity.

References

1. Faden, R.R., and Beauchamp, T.L.: A history and Theory of Informed Consent. New York, Oxford: Oxford Univ Press, 1986.

2. Faden, R.R., and Beauchamp, T.L.: Op.cit., p.3.

3. Faden, R.R., and Beauchamp, T.L.: Op.cit., pp. 39-43.

4. Griswold vs. Connecticut.

5. Pierce v. Society of Sisters. 268 U.S. 510 (1925); Loving v. Virginia, 388 U.S. 1 (1967); West Virgina State Board v. Barnette, 319 U.S. 624 (1943); Eisenstadt v. Baird, 405 U.S. 438 (1972); Roe v. Wade, 410 U.S. 113 (1973); Griswold v. Connecticut, 381 U.S. 479 (1965).

6. Schloendorff v. Society of New York Hospitals, 211 N.Y. 125, 126, 105 N.E. 92, 93 (1914).

7. In re Quinlan, 70 N.J. 10, 355 A.2d 647 (1976); In re Eichner, 52 N.Y.2d 363, 420 N.E.2d 64, 428 N.Y.S.2d 266, cert. denied, 454 U.S. 858 (1981); In re Conroy, 98 N.J. 321, 486 A.2d 1209 (1985); Bouvia v. Superior Court (Glenchur), 179 Cal. App. 3d 1127, 225 Cal. Rptr. 297 (Ct. App. 1986), review denied (Cal. JUne 5, 1986); In re Jobes, 108 N.J. 394, 529 A.2d 434 (1987); Brophy v. New England

Sinai Hospital, Inc., 398 Mass. 417, 497 N.E.2d 626 (1986).

8. Locke, J.: Of Civil Government, The Second Treatise, 1690.

9. Reck, A.: Natural Law and the Constitution. The Review of Metaphysics, 1989:483-511.

10. Kant, I.: Groundwork for the Metaphysics of Morals, Translated and analyzed by H.J. Paton. New York: Harper.

11. Kant, I.: Op.cit. p.103.

12. Kant, I.: Op.cit. p.105.

13. Kant, I.: Op.cit. p.107.

14. Hill, J.S.: On Liberty, 1859.

15. President's Commission for the Study of Ethical Problems in Medicine and Biomedical and Behavioral Research, Deciding to Forego Life-Sustaining Treatment. Washington, D.C.: March 1983.

16. Emanuel, L.L., and Emanuel, E.J.: "The Medical Directive," JAMA 1989;261:3388-93.

17. Wojtyla, K.: The Acting Person, translated from the Polish by Andrzej Potocki in collaboration with Anna-Teresa Tymieniecka. Dordrecht, Holland: Reidel, 1979.

18. Marcel, G.: Being and Having: An Existentialist Diary, translated by Katherine Farrer. New York: Harper. Pp. 172-173.

19. Pellegrino, E.D.: "Toward a Reconstruction of Medical Morality: The Primacy of the Act of Profession and the Fact of Illness." The Journal of Medicine and Philosophy 1979;4:32-56.

20. Aristotle, Politics, 1253a, 25-30.

21. Beauchamp, T.L., and McCullogh, L.B.: Medical Ethics: The Moral Responsibilities of Physicians. Englewood Cliffs, New Jersey: Prentice Hall, 1984. Pp. 82-85.

22. Pellegrino, E.D., and Thomasma, D.C.: For the

Patient's Good: The Restoration of Beneficence in Health Care. New York, Oxford: Oxford University Press, 1988.

23. Pellegrino, E.D.,: "Character, Virtue, and Self-Interest in the Ethics of the Professions,". J Comtemporary Health, Law, Policy 1989;5:53-73.

THE ROOTS OF MEDICAL ETHICS IN A SHARED MORALITY

Knut Erik Tranöy

By a shared morality I mean, in the first place, the ordinary, common, everyday morality which is, by and large, shared by the members of a given society at a given time. This **ordinary morality** I distinguish from special moralities such as medical ethics. But medical ethics is also a shared morality in a narrower sense: shared by health professionals. My focus in this paper will be on the relationship between medical ethics and ordinary morality.

There is a temptation (and not only among doctors) to regard medical ethics as, in some sense, "higher" than ordinary morality. What "higher" means here is that, in case of conflict, the principles and judgments of medical ethics take precedence over those of ordinary morality. It could also mean that doctors are bound and guided by a morality which overrides the morality of their patients because medical ethics is independent of ordinary morality.

It is my belief that today, most of us would feel that it is the other way round. If it is a question of overriding at all, it is ordinary morality which overrides medical ethics.

Thus, the thesis defended in this paper is precisely that force and acceptability of medical ethics derives from the ordinary and shared morality of the culture or society which medicine has to serve. I shall use the notions of **integrity** and **autonomy** as cases in point. But first I want to make some general comments to clarify my main thesis.

Let us first consider a human right with which we are all familiar but which is not found in the UN Declaration of Human Rights. It is the right to change one's mind. Now this may sound like a joke, and to begin with it was. In an ethics committee meeting, one of the members was criticized for abandoning a stand he had first defended. He replied, "Well, it's a human right to change one's mind". And we smiled. But the fact is - and it is not a trivial fact - that precisely in contemporary medical research ethics, the right to change one's mind has been formally institutionalized in a most striking manner. The consent form in controlled clinical trials now contains the following two points: (1) Even after having given consent, the subject is free to withdraw from the trial at any time without having to give reasons for the withdrawal. (2) In addition, there is an assurance that such withdrawal will not entail unfavorable consequences for the doctor-patient relationship of the subject. In other words, a consent to participate in a trial is not a **promise** which the subject is duty bound to keep. It is a right which means that the subjects have nothing to lose by withdrawing although the researchers may well have.

This "right to change one's mind", seldom explicitly so called, comes from general morality. It is part of what we call freedom of choice. It is also clear that it ties in with the twin ideals of integrity and autonomy, the main themes of this section. And finally it is interesting to note that this right is an ethical notion which may turn out to be more crucial and less self-evident in medical research ethics (since it has to be explicitly stated) than in ordinary morality.

There is a long history of interaction between professional medical ethics on the one hand, and moral philosophy on the other. Medical ethics is an instance of what is now often called applied ethics. This is to suggest that medical ethics is the use in practice of the theories and insights of moral philosophy. With becoming modesty, moral philosophers tend to think that, in this interaction, medical ethics has been on the receiving end. But in comtemporary biomedical ethics, it is just as much the other way round. As a brief but eloquent proof of that assertion, I quote the title of a recent paper by a well known philosopher: "How medicine saved the life of ethics" (1). It describes not only how medicine and medical ethics have contributed to the revival of interest in theoretical ethics, but also how they have given new life to ethics itself.

There is one point in particular from theoretical ethics which has been found useful by physicians concerned with ethical problems in medicine - and that is a distinction between two different kinds or types of ethics. One is consequentialist ethics, so called because it focuses mainly on what is good or bad, harmful or useful, in the consequences of our actions. The other is deontological ethics. Its distinctive feature is to regard certain actions as obligatory in themselves, as it were - it is our duty to do them regardless of their consequences. Utilitarianism is the star example of a consequentialist ethics: "the greatest good for the greatest number" is what we should aim at in our actions. Kant is the classical represenative of the other type, holding (for instance) that it is never morally right to tell a lie, no matter how bad the consequences of truthtelling, or how good the consequences of lying, are. In sum: consequentialism admonishes us to foresee and evaluate the consequences of actions. Deontological ethics looks to such things as rights and duties in the first place.

This distinction is part and parcel of ordinary morality. In our everyday lives, when choosing actions or judging those of other, we sometimes
- indeed often - look to consequences. But not always. In some cases we choose a course of action not because of its consequences but because we see it as a moral duty. Both integrity and autonomy are cases in point, and they are typically deontological notions.

Ordinary morality contains **both** kinds of principle. Some philosophers, however, have thought that we cannot have both. If consequentialism is right, then deontological ethics is wrong - and vice versa... If we accept both consequentialism and deontology, this will always generate insoluble moral conflict and contradiction. So we cannot have both utilitarianism and Kant. Ideals of consistency and rationality thus demand "a single unified moral framework" (2).

This excursion to theoretical ethics has a point relevant to our present themes.

There is no doubt that ordinary morality makes use of both, inclining in some cases more to utilitarian attitudes, in other cases more to a Kantian position. It has no definitive answer at all to the insoluble conflicts which unavoidably arise. A favorite example is "life boat ethics": discussions about who has to die when not all can be saved. They are always a mix of appeals to consequences (Not the mother of three small children!) and principles of justice and the right to live (Unfair to select **him** just because he has been in prison!). Ordinary morality has no "higher" principle to help us choose between them. But this is not seen as a reason for establishing a "single unified moral framework" by instituting as the supreme court of morality **either** some form av utilitarianism **or** some set of deontological principles.

Medical ethics follows common sense rather than philosophical sense. It is obvious that medical ethics contains both consequentialist and deontological elements - and it is difficult even to imagine that it could be otherwise. The basic aim and purpose of medicine - to fight disease and to promote health - is focused on the **consequences** of medical interventions. But it is also clear that it is non-consequentialist principles which have so radically changed the face of medical ethics - from the former profile of medical paternalism to a medical morality focusing on integrity, autonomy and patients' rights - all of them so obviously deontological notions. But in spite of the injection of rights and rights-related duties, it is as impossible as ever to imagine a medical ethics of a purely deontological kind - that is, a medical ethics which considered the consequences of medical interventions less important than obedience to a code of rules and principles. If a patient dies a death which apparently could have been prevented, it is not much of a defence if the doctor in charge replies that this was because he had simply done his duty. The only acceptable defence is that it was a consequence he, in fact but in vain, tried to prevent.

Integrity, autonomy and informed consent are frontline figures in contemporary medical ethics. And it is the notion of informed consent which offers the most convincing evidence for the insufficiency of a purely consequentialist conseption of medical ethics. Obviously, we could often secure quicker and greater gains if we did not bother about information to and consent from patients at all, and if we permitted ourselves to use prisoners, children and the mentally retarded as research subjects. But we don't – not even if the loss in terms of consequences NOT achieved is considerable: "however favorable an experiment's cost/benefit ratio might be, it is unacceptable if it involves a serious compromise of the integrity of its subjects". (3) The quotation is noteworthy because it comes from a medical ethicist who calls himself a utilitarian.

The coexistence in medical ethics of consequentialist and deontological features – which worries some philosophers – is a strength and not a weakness. Medical ethics could not be functional and realistic without this double-edged moral appeal. It does indeed create tension. But such tension is not of the nature of a contradiction, not inconsistency in an objectionable sense, as some philosophers may seem to think. The marriage – or, with a more contemporary idiom, cohabitation – of mercy and justice never was perfect harmony, but we have been able to live with that. What we cannot do is to apply the model we sometimes use in the case of logical contradictions: get rid of at least one of the two incompatible elements (4, 5). It would be absurd to suggest that, in the name of logic and order, ordinary morality has to let either justice or mercy go by the board. The statement I just quoted about the conflict between a favorable cost/benefit ratio and the integrity of research subjects is a statement of just this. Sumner, the utilitarian, is not willing to "resolve" his dilemma by giving up the principle of informed consent.

I have two more points to make on this score. One is to call attention to a noteworthy modern revival of ethical contract theories, so called. This revival also is an explicit attempt to reconcile within "a single unified moral framework" two major ethical classics – utilitarianism and Kantian moral theory (6).

The second point is that contemporary biomedical

ethics has developed and instituted new ways of managing ethical disagreements and dilemmas. Ethical committees of various kinds have become new features in familiar medical landscapes. The significance of ethical committees in our present context is their contribution to sensible decision making where moral divergence might otherwise be disruptive. They can be seen as attempts to organize rational and representative dialogues in situations the of shared common interests but diverging moral views. The aim and purpose of such dialogues whose aim and purpose is not to overcome opponents but to seek consensus.

In my concluding remarks I shall consider more closely the notions of integrity, autonomy, and informed consent. It is clear that integrity is a central notion in ordinary morality as well as in medical ethics. It is **not** clear what integrity means, and it is difficult to clarify it. An original sense of wholeness, untouchedness, and soundness is still present in it. But more central today is the ability of integrity to command unconditional respect - a respect to which any individual who is, has been, or could have been an autonomous human person is entitled. A human person is a union of a human body and a human mind. For some purposes it may be useful to distinguish between mental and physical (or bodily) integrity. But that distinction does not seem to be as important as the quality of commanding respect for the basic and equal dignity and moral worth of persons - so understood that (for instance) the mentally retarded are entitled to no less respect than the rest of us, and the very intelligent to no more.

Within the domains of western culture, a medical ethics which openly violated or denied the integrity of persons could not now be a viable medical ethics.

I also think that integrity could not be a viable ideal in contemporary medicine if it were not in the first place a well entrenched ideal in our shared ordinary morality.

What does "well entrenched" mean here? It means, for one thing, that integrity is strongly and intimately linked with certain other moral notions and ideals which are widely accepted in our Western culture: **autonomy** and **informed consent** in the first place. These three are occupying strikingly central positions and roles in contemporary medical ethics.

And this was not always so.

This also means that we cannot say <u>yes</u> to one (or two) of these three and say <u>no</u> to the third. If somebody said, "Yes, I accept that you have autonomy but I will not let you make your own decisions", he would be in moral conflict with himself. It is quite possible to see this without necessarily also seeing what precisely the consept of integrity means.

It seems reasonable to say that the informed consent requirement follows from, or is instrumental to, the other two. We know, indeed, that informed consent is a very difficult notion to handle, in theory as in practice. But to simply abandon the attempt to implement **some** kind of informed consent would amount to a rejection of integrity (respect for persons) and autonomy (moral self-determination) as moral values.

The more difficult part of the question concerns the relationship between integrity and autonomy. They are not identical notions. Integrity seems to be, morally speaking, the more fundamental of the two. A key to an understanding of it may be found in Kant's Categorical imperative, especially that version of it which forbids us to use human persons as a means only. (Kant's demand that we should also treat them as ends in themselves may likewise be understood as the right to pursue self-chosen goals provided such pursuit does not violate "the moral law".)

Integrity, I said, seems morally more basic than autonomy. Evidence of this is the fact that autonomy admits of degrees, in contrast to integrity. A person's autonomy can be reduced or constrained or annihilated by inner or outer circumstances.

Integrity is not a function of intellectual abilities such as intelligence. But autonomy is. And the range of a person's integrity extends beyond the boundary of death.

In the West, the moral entrenchment of integrity has been taken to mean also that the rights of human persons should take precedence over the rights and needs of society. In other words, as we now understand it, it means that society cannot legitimately use the individual merely as a means to greater collective welfare. It is this understanding of the ideal of integrity which has been given such prominent recognition in the Helsinki Declaration of the World Medical Association: "concern for the interests of the subject must always prevail over the interests of science and society".

That is a very firm constraint on the free search for knowledge in a culture where such search is regarded as the foundation of almost any kind of human welfare.

I have argued that a workable medical ethics must have its roots in the norm and value systems of a shared ordinary morality. This means that it must also adjust to the moral, cultural, and religious heritage of the society it has to serve.

But is not this really to **undermine** the validity of medical - and any other - ethics? Is not this to let **moral and cultural relativism** in by the front door?

This IS a challenge, and it is my conviction that it should be met head on. Of course, there are forms of relativism, cultural and moral, which are unacceptable. They should, indeed, be defeated when they amount to arbitrary subjectivism or cultural chauvinism. It IS unacceptable relativism to say and believe that the moral view which I hold, or **my** society holds, is right, and for that reason. I hope it is clear that the picture I have tried to draw of medical ethics in interaction with ordinary morality is not threatened by such relativism and subjectivism. On the contrary, I have stressed the importance of a representative and rational dialogue in the management of moral disagreement and dilemmas, especially in medical ethics. **That** is to treat moral diversity as a resource and not as a scandal.

There was a time not so long ago when we all (?) were impressed and frightened by the prospects of cultural relativism. More recent insights - the revival of a normative applied ethics - should have allayed some of those fears. I think we are now in a position to see that there can be no validity and functional viability for **any** morality without a cultural anchorage, that is to say, without roots in the cultural and moral traditions of a living society. There must, of course, be limits to this kind of relativism. The limits are set by the scope of shared and common interests and values. Medicine and medical science define a very wide ranging community in this sense. And no ethics, I am sure, can claim validity or be workable where there is no longer, in some sense, community.

References

1. Toulmin, S.E.: How medicine saved the life of ethics. Perspectives in Biology and Medicine, 1982;25:736-50.

2. Sumner, L.W.: Utilitarian Goals and Kantian Constraints. In: Brody, B.A. (ed.) Moral Theory and Moral Judgments in Medical Ethics. Dordrecht: Kluwer Academic Publishers, 1988, p.18.

3. Sumner, L.W.: In Brody (ed.) op.cit. p.17.

4. Tranöy, K.E. Biomedical Value Conflict. In: Jones, A.J.I. (ed.) The Moral Import of Science. Bergen: Sigma Forlag, 1988;18:98-107.

5. Tranöy, K.E.: In: Hastings Center Report 1988; 18:No 4.

6. Rawls, J.: A Theory of Justice. Cambridge, Mass.: Harvard University Press, 1971.

Ethics in Medicine, edited by
Peter Allebeck and Bengt Jansson.
Raven Press, New York © 1990.

INTEGRITY AND AUTONOMY FROM AN ANTHROPOLOGICAL POINT OF VIEW

Lisbeth Sachs

Introduction

My role here is to discuss integrity and autonomy from an anthropological point of view. I shall try to convey how an anthropological perspective helps to even further complicate what we are talking about in medical ethics. The strength of the interpretive approach in anthropological work is that, although the researcher records an account of the beliefs and actions of other people, the exercise is done with an awareness that the interpretation is itself a product of particular historical and cultural determinants. Ideally, no assumption should be made that any analytical viewpoint is value free. But the notion of total relativism could be quite paralyzing and the relativistic thinking should preferably be used as a method in analytical work. When combined with rich and detailed descriptive data, this type of work has furnished us with invaluable possibilities for cross cultural comparisons and holds up a mirror in which to see ourselves. With this in mind I want to share my perspective and look at such concepts as integrity and autonomy in the context of culture. First a few words about what I mean by culture.

Cultures, including those of industrial-capitalistic societies like Sweden, form systems of meanings which provide explanations of how the world works, of what is thought of as real and what is designated as natural and inevitable as well as what is morally right. These meanings link people to one another and form the basis for social action. One can look upon the treating of bodily ills in any culture, as an action that takes place within a metamedical framework of thought. This framework can be looked upon as an overarching philosophy which guides the basic features of medical knowledge, its organization and practice, within which moral codes and ethical principles are in use. It is thus within this framework that the boundaries for integrity and autonomy of any person are considered in situations of health care.

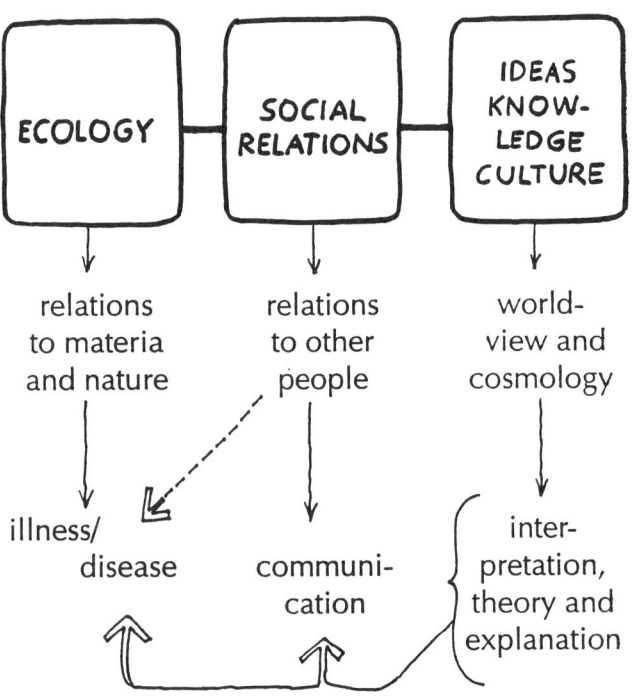

Let us look at the model in Fig. 1 of the inter-relationship between materia, people and their ideas. It is within such a world of experience that concepts like integrity and autonomy get their content and meaning.

Human beings build up their understanding of the world in relationships to other beings with whom they share their environment and similar conditions for survival (ecology). There is a constant process in which meanings are being created by people in their relations to other people wherever they live. When things happen that scare or threaten the group, theories and explanations follow. Whether these explanations are folk or scientific in nature, they help people to cope with reality and their everyday life. This is of course also true of reactions to illness and death.

Like all systems of healing, biomedicine is a cultural product; it is formed in, reflects, and helps to create and recreate a social and cultural world (1). Biomedicine must be understood in its cultural context. Bodies of medical knowledge and accompanying practices are symbolic systems: they have referents to other aspects of culture beyond their ostensible boundaries. Although diseases have biological correlates, how they are recognized (if at all), expressed as illness, classified, understood, valued, and treated varies greatly from culture to culture (2, 3). Biomedicine, like all other medical systems, reflects the dominant characteristics of the culture of which it is a part.

Illness/disease is an event that challenges meaning in life. Medical beliefs and practices organise the event into an episode that gives it form and meaning. Cosmologies are above all means of explaining, predicting and attempting to control the relationship between the individual and his or her society.

Individual versus society and the notion of body-self

The significance of such concepts as integrity and autonomy in other worlds, as in our own, is often a reflection of the relationship between the individual and society and the notion of what we may call the body-self (4).

The relation of individual to society, which has

occupied so much of contemporary social theory, is based on a perceived natural opposition between the demands of the social and moral order on the one hand, and egocentric drives, impulses, wishes, and needs on the other. The individual/society opposition, while fundamental to Western epistemology, is also rather particular to it. The wellknown anthopologist Clifford Geerts (5) has argued that the Western conception of the person "as a bounded, unique... integrated motivational and cognitive universe, a dynamic center of awareness, emotion, judgement, and action is a rather peculiar idea within the context of the world's cultures". In fact, the modern conception of the individual self is of recent historical origin, even in the West.

It may be a reasonable assumption that all humans have some selfconsciousness of mind and body, with some kind of internal body image, but it is important to distinguish this universal awareness of the individual body-self from the social conception of the individual as person, a construct of jural rights and moral accountability. The Western notion of the individual as a quasi-sacred, legal, moral and psychological entity, whose rights are limited by the rights of other equally autonomous individuals, is unique.

In Japan for example, it is the family which is considered the most natural fundamental unit of society, not the individual. In general, Japan has been repeatedly described as a culture in which the person is understood as acting within the context of a social relationship, never simply autonomously. One's self-identity changes with the social context, particularly within the hierarchy of social relations at any given time.

Another example is a society in New Guinea where people lack a concept of the person altogether. Individual identity and social identity are two sides of the same coin (6). Such sociocentric conceptions of the self have been widely documented for many parts of the world and have relevance to ethnomedical understanding. In cultures and societies lacking a highly individualized or articulated conception of the body-self it should not be surprising that sickness is often explained in terms of such social relations as sorcery, or to the breaking of social and moral codes, or to disharmony within the family or the village community. In such a society, therapy too, tends to be collective.

In contrast to societies in which the individual body-self tends to be fused with or absorbed by the social body, there are societies that view the individual as comprised of a multiplicity of selves. The Bororo in Africa understand the individual only as reflected in relation to other people. Hence, the person consists of many selves - the self as perceived by parents, by other kinsmen, by enemies etc. The Cuna Indians of Panama say they have eight selves, each associated with a different part of the body. A Mayan community in Mexico states that the soul has 13 divisible parts. Each time a person loses one or more parts, he or she becomes ill and a curing ceremony is held to retrieve the missing pieces. At death the soul leaves the body and returns to where it came from - a soul depository kept by the ancestral gods. This soul pool is used for the creation of new human beings, each of whose own soul is made up of 13 parts from the life-force of other previous humans. A person's soul-force and his or her self, is therefore a composite from many other humans. There is no sense in which each man is a brand new or unique individual; rather each person is a fraction of the whole social world (7).

In our industrialized world, states in which a person experiences more than one self are invariably explained as pathological (as in schizophrenia). In many non-Western cultures individuals can experience multiple selves through the normative practice of spirit possession and other altered states of consciousness.

For most people the body, the human organism and its natural products of blood, milk, tears, semen and excreta may be used as a cognitive map to represent other natural, supernatural, social and even spatial relations. The body is a natural symbol supplying some of our richest sources of metaphor (7). Particular organs, body fluids, and functions may also have special significance to a group of people. We know that the liver carries a great deal of blame for different ailments among the French. The English and the Germans are by comparison far more obsessed with the condition and health of their bowels (8, 9). Blood is a nearly universal symbol of human life and some peoples, both ancient and contemporary, have taken the quality of the blood, pulse and circulation as the primary diagnostic sign of health or illness.

The concept of blood has been analyzed as a predominant metaphor in European culture, especially its use in political ideologies, as during the Nazi era. Similarly the multiple stigma suffered by aids patients include a preoccupation with bad blood (10). But where one society would extract bad blood, another would feel blood does not regenerate and should therefore not be tapped (11).

That the body is so rich in metaphors may of course also mean that certain parts or fluids are more or less valuable to people and more or less tabu. The body as a part of cosmos or as a symbol of integrity causes people in various parts of the world to regard an autopsy or a transplan as exotic, barbarian or absolutely impossible. In short, what we can call ethno-anatomical perceptions, including body image, offer a rich source of data both on the social and cultural meanings of being human and on the various threats to health, well-being, and social integration that humans are believed to experience.

In our modern biomedicine the body and self are understood as distinct and separable entities; illness resides in either the body or the mind or the one may impose illness on the other, what we call psychosomatic states. By contrast, many ethnomedical systems do not logically distinguish body, mind and self, and therefore illness cannot be situated in mind or body alone. Social relations with the living and the dead are there understood as key contributors to individual health and illness. Illness and death can be attributed to social tensions, contradictions, and hostilities, as manifested in the hot cold syndrome and symptomatic imbalance in various folk medicines and in such folk idioms as withcraft or the evil eye. Each of these beliefs exemplifies the link between the health or illness of the individual body and the social body.

Let us look at how two medical systems approach the diseased person and start from the following example.

WESTERN MEDICAL MICROSYSTEM

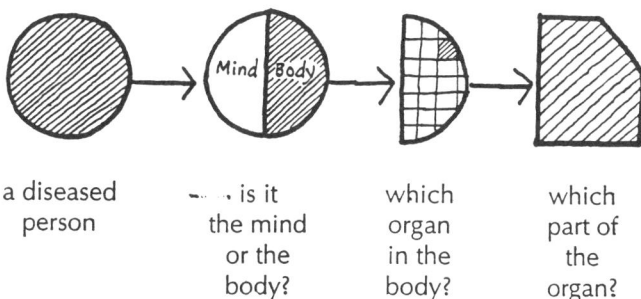

| a diseased person | → is it the mind or the body? | which organ in the body? | which part of the organ? |

NON-WESTERN MEDICAL MACROSYSTEM

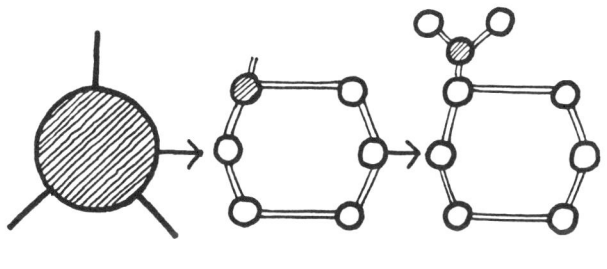

a diseased person — which relations to the living are disturbed? — which relations to the dead ancestors are disturbed?

(Borgå 1983)

In this non-Western system (actually an African society) the body is seen as a unitary, integrated aspect of self and social relations (12). It is dependent on, and vulnerable to, the feelings, wishes, and actions of others, including spirits and dead ancestors. The body is perceived as a microcosm of the universe and not as a complex machine, whose every detail may be manipulated or even exchanged as is the case in the Western macro-system. On top we see the Western system, where the body is an independent entity and the search for disease causes is concentrated on more and more physical detail.

These systems of medical ideas give people a structure of how to feel, how to communicate and how to explain illness. Thus the structure of individual and collective sentiments, down to the feel of one's body and the naturalness of one's position and role in the order of things, is a social and cultural construct. Non-industrialized people think of the world with their bodies. They exercise their power by naming the phenomena and creatures of the world in their own image and likeness. We in the West live in a world in which the humans shape things and even themselves, with mechanical hearts and plastic hips. While the cosmologies of non-industrialized people speak of a constant exchange of metaphors from body to nature and back to body again, our metaphors often speak of machine to body symbolic equations (13).

What does all this mean for our concern with integrity and autonomy in health care? Well, if we look at the major differences between some non-Western perceptions of the body-self, and our own notion of what is a person, we may be able to problematize health care over cultural boundaries in a new way.

The encounter

When confronted with people who do not share our cosmology we are often at a loss to understand their inner world of experience. We have difficulties to see what integrity and autonomy may mean to them. In my own research among a group of peasant Turkish migrants in Sweden (11) I have experienced their cosmology as a structure of supernatural agencies with quite different principles of responsibility for misfortune, illness and death, than those existing in Swedish health care today. These families have systematic explanations of personal misfortune which involve the notion of destiny or the will and power of other external powers, which means that the individual alone cannot be responsible for illness or any other misfortune. As we can understand, an appeal to individual responsibility in the prevention or control of illness will have a different meaning and different effect among this group of people.

When the Turkish women came to Sweden from their villages, they brought with them the experience of an ecology quite different from the suburbs of Stockholm. They had a view of life and death which differed from ours in several ways. They were used to children often dying at birth or soon after. (According to some statistics, the child mortality rate was up to 20 percent in some of their villages). Of course this situation elicited theories and explanations. The women believed in external and evil beings that threatened their children; but the ultimate explanation was that God took the children so that they could prepare for their parents when they died. Also the elderly women told about how their parents had decided when they wanted to die, said good-bye to their families, and died. The belief in a life after life on earth, and the expectations that children may die at birth, made their reactions to specific experiences in Sweden strange from a Swedish point of view.

With Sweden's advanced medical technology, almost all children are saved at birth no matter what physical complication or injury they may have. The women from Anatolia were taken by surprise that the Swedes did not let the children die - they could even oppose what might be the will of God. One woman also exclaimed that children born in Sweden seemed to have "an inferior quality" to the children she had seen in her own village. Some kinds of handicap that children survived with in Sweden had never existed where she came from, where, of course, as in many parts of the world, complications at birth mean death. It is also in line with this puzzlement from the women's point of view that they sometimes left handicapped children with Swedish institutions. The children were not within the boundaries of what they knew as normal and therefore they belonged to God. So the people who opposed God's will, the Swedes, should take care of the child.

Since every death had a logical explanation having to do with destiny or the power or will of other beings or God, the women never felt any guilt or responsibility in connection with illness or death. They felt they were a part of a larger order where they just had to follow their fate.

Communication in health care

Let me finally talk about the actual communication

of messages in everyday health care encounters between patients and practitioners who do not share a common background and mutual expectations. It is within such encounters that medical personnel often experience an enormous strain, having to deal with what they see as quite different patients. The problems in such encounters are often looked upon and critically described as arising from the doctors' ignorance of folkconcepts of illness, but also from the asymmetrical medical relationships and the doctors' attitude of superiority.

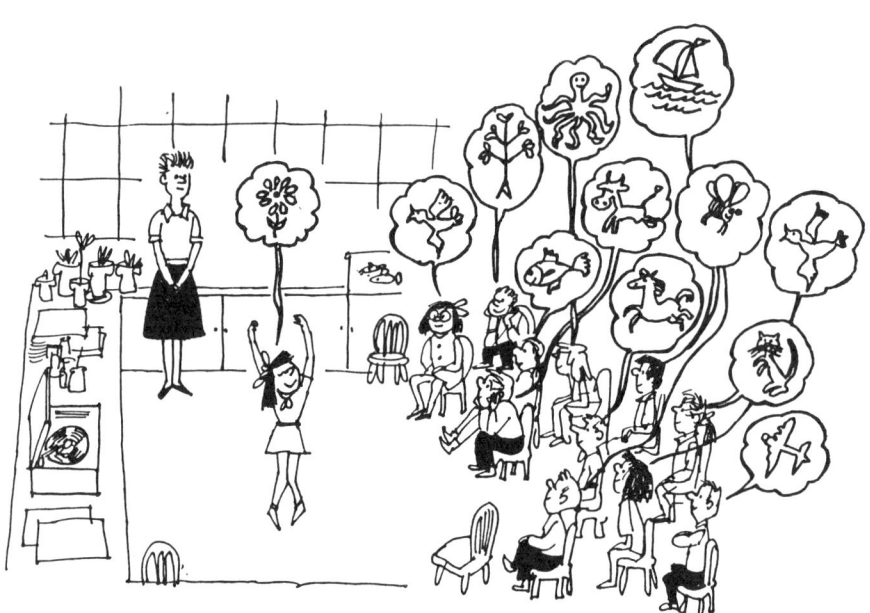

I would like to take the opportunity to approach and problematize some of this critique. I shall do so by using a small illustration. The picture illustrates a common situation when people communicate with each other. Let's look at the situation as one where the girl with the flower is a patient from another culture. She communicates her symptoms with help of a symbolic language which is hers. The various health care personnel, sitting to the right in the picture, understand her message in their own way. They understand her language of symptoms through <u>their</u> world of experience. Since they are more or less secure in their interpretation of what the patient means, and thus what is her problem, they also treat her as if they have understood what it was *she* means. And this may proceed without any of the persons involved noticing that the pictures they have of each others' messages are not the same.

This example may be provocative, but my point is that in most communication people never really know whether they have understood what the other person meant. They do not normally question their own interpretations. My experience of communication in health care over cultural boundaries fits this description quite well.

Both in the research I have done in Sri Lanka (14) and among the Turkish migrants in Sweden it has been obvious that Western biomedical care is seen in an entirely different way by the Sinalese and Turkish patients than among their practitioners. In the Sri Lankan case the Sinhalese, Buddhist patients have integrated Western medicines/drugs into their thinking about the body, illness and therapy. The Western medicines that the practitioners prescribe for what they judge as well-defined diseases, are being used by the patients according to what they perceive as a hot or cold quality; a red pill may thus be used as a hot medicine against what they see as a cold disease. They interprete disease as evidence of imbalance in their relations to cosmos, to nature, to other people or between fluids in the body and use the Western medicines to restore an equilibrium. The mutual (but different) confidence that practitioners and patients have in the medicines, helps prevent the misinterpretations of each other's beliefs from being discovered. They don't question the ongoing interaction. Health care seems to work not only despite their respective misinterpretations but also because of them.

Most native Swedes expect regular medical care to include verbal consultation and communication around existential matters having to do with health. Many of our migrants, as well as people in other parts of the world, have expectations of a more technical kind, partly because they have other options for social and existential kinds of problems but also because they seem to have a realistic view of what biomedicine can give them. Such expectations are readily met and often lead to satisfaction. Both doctors and patients may be satisfied with what is going on but on different grounds.

Let me give one short example to make this clear: the peasant women who came from villages in Turkey were used to folkhealers. Among other methods these healers wrote amulets; sacred words on small pieces of paper folded and sewn into a piece of cloth. The illiterate women used the power of the words in the amulet as their medicine, put it in water which they then drank, or burnt it and inhaled the smoke. Some women used the prescription they got from Swedish physicians in the same way; put it into a glass of water and drank the water. They said they had been healed by the medicine and the doctors got confirmation that they had prescribed correctly.

Our dilemma in such cases is that as long as we do not know that we don't understand each other "properly" or know exactly what the other means, the problem is not revealed. But as soon as we understand that we do not know what the other actor means, we have the whole responsibility to make this clear. There is obviously more satisfaction when encounters in health care are built on unknown misinterpretations than when they are built on known misinterpretations. Furthermore much of the positive placebo effects in health care are retained when the patient and the doctor think they understand each other.

All this may sound cynical, but we must accept that although communication in everyday health care often resembles this picture, much of its outcome is quite satisfactory. Such concepts as informed consent and the autonomy and integrity of the patient might be less dramatic if looked at with an understanding that misinterpretation often works. What, by the way, is a perfect understanding of what a life, good health, a normal body or death means to a person from another world of experience?

Complicated life-threatening situations must, however, be dealt with situationally and with the help of ethical rules and the law. But this is true with any patient, be it a Swedish Jehova's witness who refuses blood transfusion to a dying child, or a Muslim tribal woman from Africa who wants a circumcision made so that she will be an accepted part of her social group and not unclean.

We may feel that a utilitarian philosophy works quite well within a given culture. It uses the greatest happiness principle to provide directions about rational choice when the consequences of an action are knowable and the values agreed. Between two alternatives, it says choose the one which is expected to yield the greatest happiness to the greatest number. Its decisions depend upon knowing the consequences and knowing what will give happiness. Where the consequences are uncertain it gives no guidance. Where tastes and values are uncertain it retreats to those that seem more certain, so it tends to focus on the material wants, the common need of food and shelter for mere survival, or medicines for the priority of life and health. We can take the resulting materialist trend for granted, if we stay within our own culture. But once we start to compare judgements of happiness in a cultural prespective, we see that in some moral systems happiness is not reducible to the conditions of survival. Sometimes the manner of dying is valued more highly than living, sometimes to live courting death is more valued than living safely. Some cultures make a call to heroism that is quite outside the purview of the greatest happiness principle. The guidance of utilitarian ethics depends on knowable consequences, and we are in a society in which technological change is so swift that consequences cannot be known. We must accept that we are part of a socially pluralist world, so values over cultural boundaries cannot often be agreed.

My ambition has been to discuss integrity and autonomy in their cultural contexts. I have also ventured to take up the problem of meaning in communication over cultural boundaries. I have argued that misinterpretations in human communication are more often a rule than an exception. That migrants may feel they preserve their integrity and autonomy in health care in Sweden is therefore often a result of undiscovered mis-interpretations made by them and their practitioners, rather than a result of their joint understanding of meaning and value.

References

1. Hepburn, S.J.: Western minds, foreign bodies. Medical Anthropology Quaterly 1988;2:59-74.

2. Comaroff, J.: The defectiveness or symbols, or the symbols of defectiveness? Culture, Medicine and Psychiatry 1983;7:3-20.

3. Kleinman, A.: Medicine's symbolic reality: On a central problem in the philosophy of medicine.

Inquiry 1973;16:206-221.

4. Scheper-Hughes, N., and Lock, M.M.: The mindful body: A prolegomenon to future work in medical anthropology. Medical Anthropology Quaterly 1987;1:6-41.

5. Geertz, C.: From the native's point of view: On the nature of anthropological understanding. In Culture Theory. R. Shweder and R. LeVine, eds. Cambridge:Cambridge University Press. 1984:123-136.

6. Read, K.E.: Morality and the concept of the person among the Guhuku-Gama. Oceania 1955;25:233-282.

7. Douglas, M.: Natural symols. New York: Vintage. 1970.

8. Dundes, A.: Life is like a chicke-coop ladder. New York: Columbia, University Press. 1984.

9. Miller, J.: The body in question. Ney Work: Vintage. 1978.

10. Lancaster, R.G.: What AIDS is doing to us. Christopher Street 1983;7:48-52.

11. Sachs, L.: Evil eye or bacteria: Turkish migrant women and Swedish health care. Stockholm studies in social anthropology series, SSSA No 12, University of Stockholm, Stockholm, Sweden. 1983.

12. Borgå, P.: Traditional medicine versus western psychology and psychiatry (in Swedish). Social-medicinsk Tidskrift 1983;60:7.

13. O'Neill, J.: Five bodies: The human shape of modern society. Ithaca: Cornell University Press. 1985.

14. Sachs, L.: Misunderstanding as therapy: Doctors, patients and medicines in a rural clinic in Sri Lanka. Culture, Medicine and Psychiatry. 1989;13:335-349.

Ethics in Medicine, edited by
Peter Allebeck and Bengt Jansson.
Raven Press, New York © 1990.

THE IDEAS OF INTEGRITY AND AUTONOMY: DISCUSSION

Erwin Bischofberger

The task I have been given for this paper is to review and discern the previous authors' reflections on integrity and autonomy. In order to save time I have chosen to give a summary of what has been said in combination with my own commentaries. I am in other words not presenting a collection of specific quotations from already presented papers. I am trying to approach my task in three steps, with some remarks at the end.

The concepts

Let us take the first step by asking how we can define the concepts of integrity and autonomy. Searching for the etymological roots integrity has its origin in the latin term <u>integritas</u> which means wholeness, completeness, coherence, harmony. The ancient romans imagined an integral person to be coherent in character and consistent in behaviour. They also imagined an integral system, e.g. the human body, to be and to function as a wholeness where the parts belong and attribute to the completeness and harmony of the system.

Autonomy has its roots in the greek term <u>autonomia</u> which means self-determination and independence. The greek city-state of Athens (the polis) was regarded to be independent on other comparable political units. Also a free citizen, but not a slave, was autonomous.

It is important to note that both the <u>idea</u> integrity and autonomy in antiquity were treated as ethical terms.

When we try to translate the ideas of integrity and autonomy into the ethical discussion of our time we find ourselves right in the heart of the meaning of ethics. Both ideas indicate what ethics is all about. We still hear an echo of the etymological origins of the term when we give the following definition of the concept: Integrity signifies the moral value of wholeness, (1) constituting all human beings as persons and ends in themselves, independent on all functions, and (2) demanding respect for their dignity and moral worth. The concept of integrity indicates thus a fundamental notion of the concept of man.

The concept of autonomy also indicates some echo of its original meaning: Autonomy signifies the moral principle of self-determination, (1) depending on cognitive and voluntary functions of a competent person, and (2) responding to the moral demand of respect for all persons' integrity. Whereas the concept of integrity is designed to express a fundamental value equivalent to the dignity of the human person, the concept of autonomy expresses the idea of an action guideline, a principle of action directed towards safeguarding and promoting the highest and most fundamental value, namely the integrity of each person.

The definitions I have given the concepts of integrity and autonomy may probably be traced back to the papers of both professor Pellegrino och professor Tranöy.

<u>The properties</u>

Let us then take our second step by asking what the specific properties of the concepts of integrity and autonomy are. While the concept of integrity includes and concerns all persons the concept of autonomy includes only conscious persons who are capable to express their will. The integrity of a person can be violated and lost. The value of integrity admits of no degrees and is consequently invariable whereas he power and principle of autonomy admits of degrees and is variable. A small child, a professor in biotechnology or bioethics and a senile patient have all the same integrity and the same claim on respect for their integrity, but they have not the same amount of autonomy. The integrity of a person is constantly the same, it is by contrast the degree of autonomy which increases and diminishes.

It is then consistent to affirm that the integrity of a person never can be substituted by any proxy decision. Integrity can be respected or violated, but never substituted. It is the weakened or lost autonomy of a person or patient that can and must be substituted by proxy decisions. The weaker the autonomy of a person has become the more it must be substituted in order to secure and promote his/her integrity.

There is still another, most important property which must be expounded here and which more than everything else can reveal the innermost meaning of what we want to express with the ideas of integrity and autonomy. Professor Pellegrino and I myself have quite independently - autonomously if you wish- expressed the idea that whereas integrity indicates a value on the level of <u>being</u> and identity, autonomy indicates a principle on the level of <u>doing</u> or action. Without having any intention of doing harm to anybody we can observe that we in our western industrialised and technified civilisations give preference to autonomy and action and tend to neglect the integrity of mainly the weak and helpless and dependent groups of human beings. We live in a social context where what we are depends on what we do. Experiences and feelings of selfrespect and identity are rooted in what we do and not in what we are. During the Middle Ages it was a common axiom that doing was anchored in being (agere sequitur esse). Today it is the other way round which I suggest is not to the advantage of our time. In restoring the fundamental value of integrity we can find ourselves on the threshold to a culture that hopefully again will give priority to being before doing.

<u>The application</u>

We take the third step by applying the notions of

integrity and autonomy in the concrete "clinical workshop" where the problems of informed consent are an everyday experience of physicians and nurses. Roughly speaking we have three categories of patients. The first category has both integrity and autonomy. They are competent patients. A large number of for example cancer patients, gynecology and ortopedic patients would belong to this category. They have retained the power of decision making. The second category of patients have lost or not yet obtained autonomy but are in possession of the same integrity as the first category. Here we should find all embryos, small children, unconscious, senile and heavily psychotic patients. Relatives and caregivers must substitute the lacking autonomy in order to secure the patients' integrity.

The third category of patients would from the ethical point of view be the most interesting and the most difficult group. They are human beings or patients on the way to full possession of autonomy or, on the opposite side of man's life span, on the way out of an autonomous way of life. In this group we find older children, roughly between 10 and 18 years with varying degrees of autonomy. How much autonomy should they be allowed to exercise, how much support do they need, how much should their autonomy be substituted? Is a 15 years old girl demanding abortion able to make an autonomous decision, must her demand for secrecy be respected? In Sweden the law recognizes full autonomy when a person has become 18 years old. For patients before that age the doctor must decide the degree of autonomy in each single case.

My point was to show that while patients have various degrees of autonomy they are in possession of one and the same integrity. The less autonomy a patient has the more his integrity must be maintained. Here we can ask the question who in our modern societies are the most helpless, the most exposed human beings whose integrity is most threatened. Probably many immigrants who according to professor Sachs have their own value systems become alienated in another value system where they cannot exercise their autonomy because they are not understood. Their integrity is easily violated.

Some years ago a well known professor of medicine in Sweden said at a conference: "The integrity of an embryo is almost equal to zero." We understand now that he of course should have said that what was almost zero was the autonomy of the embryo, and not his integrity. It is essential to make the right distinctions and to choose the right words.

I am heading toward the end of my short paper with a couple of remarks. When I in the spring term of 1984 studied at Georgetown (with the help of professor Pellegrino) I asked professor Tom Beauchamp what his idea of integrity was. He answered me that to his notion integrity rather meant a virtue than a value. His answer has made me think that there might be a small difference in the American and European ethical thought. But today professor Pellegrino has made a great impression on me for his strong defence of the fundamental value of integrity.

Since 1982 we have a new health care law in Sweden. In its opening paragraph the law says that medical care must be built on the respect for the patient's self-determination and integrity. The law does not define the concept of integrity and does not attempt to describe any distinction between self-determination and integrity. There is in my experience a vast uncertainty and a great confusion among caregivers, both doctors and nurses and social workers, as to what the two ideas mean. I think that today's reflections have been necessary and useful. I hope that they have attributed to fill this gap and to clarify a very interesting field in general ethics and in specific medical ethics.

Let me conclude by saying that since 1973, when I came to Stockholm, I have tried to articulate a common base of communication and a ground of shared values. This has been quite an exciting work which we continue in the National Medical Ethics Council. There the ideas of both integrity and autonomy have an important place, but first integrity, and then autonomy.

PRIORITIES IN MEDICAL HEALTH CARE

INTRODUCTION

Gösta Gahrton

Setting priorities has always been part of the decision-making process in medicine. The rapidly increasing possibilities to treat diseases with highly specialized technology as well as the increase of the aged population has focused the attention on the priority problem. I most societies, resources are lacking for giving all patients immediate, optimal treatment for any disorder. Thus lining-up for treatment like hip replacement, cataract treatment, coronary by-pass, etc., is an increasingly common phenomenon. For the political decision makers, the level of priority is how to allocate the limited resources and how to handle the ever-increasing requests from the medical profession and patient groups. For the medical profession, prioritizing in the ward or in the admittance room for emergencies is a delicate and difficult task. Should priorities be set on the level of individual patients or on the level of patient groups. Should the patient with the most severe disease or with the disease that is most likely to be cured by the treatment available be treated first?

Another important issue is how to inform patients and the public about the necessity of setting priorities. Do the politicians and the medical profession agree about how to inform about the lack of resources, and how this lack of resources affects the possibility to use the best possible treatment? In fact, there are many indications that politicians frequently underestimate the problems when informning the public. Sweeping statements like "every patient will be treated with the best available methods" or "economic reasons will never go before the health of the people" are common.

This section will deal with the ethical aspects of setting priorities. It will focus both on the use of highly specialized, costly technology and on other aspects, such as age as a limiting factor in the process of setting priorities.

Ethics in Medicine, edited by
Peter Allebeck and Bengt Jansson.
Raven Press, New York © 1990.

SETTING LIMITS IN HEALTH CARE

Daniel Callahan

There can be little doubt that the triumphs of biological knowledge, and of biomedical research and application, are among the greatest of all human achievements. They have greatly lengtened the average human life span, have cured a whole range on once-lethal infectious diseases and have significantly relieved us of the burden of many serious illnesses and disabilities. They have led us to expand the role of medicine, to broaden our understanding of health and, perhaps most importantly, have led us to think differently about our lives as human beings. Illness, injury, and death are still great threats, but our chances of living to an old age in reasonably good health are extraordinarily high. The risks of life have been reduced, the possibilities of human flourishing increased. That is indeed a remarkable achievement.

The question I want to examine here is just how much further, and in what way, we can continue to pursue that progress. If there can be little doubt about the past achievements of biomedicine, there is also little reason to doubt the possibility of still more such achievements in the future. The French philosopher Condorcet in 1795 spoke of the "unlimited progress" that was possible for medicine, and he has yet to be proved wrong.

Yet a cloud has appeared on that bright, optimistic horizon of "unlimited progress", in fact more than one cloud. Two of them are particularly noticeable. The first is that not everything that represents a medical advance is necessarily "progress", that is, it may not genuinely better our human condition even if it represents a scientific development. The most obvious and widespread general example of this phenomenon is that of the declining rates of mortality and the increasing rates of chronic illness. We live longer but also with a greater burden of illness as a consequence. Despite some scientific optimism about the eventual eradication of chronic illness - especially cancer, heart disease, and stroke - only in the case of heart disease is any actual decline apparent. Nor is there any solid evidence yet to support the hope that, while life may not be greatly extended in the future, a compression of morbidity prior to death will occur.

The second cloud is represented by the rising costs of contemporary medical care, costs that have begun to place a great strain on the finances of the developed countries, and particularly the United States, which now devotes 11.3% of its Gross National Product to health care. The reasons for these rising costs have been much debated, but the principal candidates appear to be three: an aging population, increased use of technological medicine with that population, and a steady increase in public demand for good, state-of-the-art medical care. An aging population is itself not necessarily a cause of increasing costs; it is instead what economists in the United States call an "intensification of services" for that population, most notably a greater use of high-technology medicine. A reported five-fold increase in surgical procedures for those over the age of 90 at the famous Mayo Clinic in the past decade is, perhaps, an extreme example of this phenomenon but hardly an isolated one.

What we have come to discover, then, is that medical progress, particularly progress with an aging population and in the face of pervasive chronic illness, is a very expensive matter - and is likely to become even more so in the future, as the proportion of elderly grows and as new technologies to extend and improve life continue to be developed. What are we to do about this problem? A common and popular response in the United States is that a more efficient health care system, one less wasteful of resources, can well cope with the expected strains in the future. I will call this the economic solution, meaning by that a solution which would not change any fundamental values about the desirability of "indefinite progress", but would look to careful organization, planning, technology assessment and suitable patient and provider incentives to get us through the coming years.

I do not believe it makes sense any longer to continue looking exclusively to an economic solution. There are no inherent limits to the possibility of spending an unlimited amount of money on unlimited medical progress on the frontiers of medicine. We can <u>hope</u> to find inexpensive solutions, or cures for chronic illness, and a compression of morbidity. But it does not make sense to base policy on hope; instead, policy should be based on a sober assessment of the future based on what we now know, not what we would like to be the case.

In that respect, the available information, and reasonable future projections, indicate that the economic solutions will and must fail. We will have to change some fundamental values, and be prepared to live with a less ambitious view of medical progress, and a less soaring vision of the liberation of human beings from illness, decline, and death. What I will call the philosophical view, then, will emphasize a shift in our values, our hopes, and our expectations. We will have both to adopt all of the economist's recommendations and, at the same time, change our values as well. In pressing for a change in values, I am not, therefore, arguing that we do not need, or that they are useless, what the economists propose. I am simply arguing that their approach will not be sufficient. It must be supplemented by some profound changes in our thinking.

I approach this complicated task with the image in mind of an implosion. How can we turn the explosive force and intensity of our quest for improved health inward rather than always outward? I suggest we can begin thinking about this possibility by means of the image of restricting exploration on the two great frontiers of medicine, that of aging and that of individual cure.

1. Setting Limits: Aging and Individual Need

A system that seeks implosion rather than explosion must, above all, admit of firm limits. That acceptance of limits should build upon some basic, undeniable truths of human existence. The most important of these is that the human body is finite. It is part of its nature to become ill, to age, and eventually to die. At its best - now and forever- medicine can only forestall death and relieve for a time, and only that, the diseases and frailties of the body. An appropriate and prudent goal for medicine is to provide a reasonably healthy life within the framework and limitations of a human life that is, of its nature, finite and bounded. An obsessive pursuit of health, an unwillingness to accept death, and a never-ending struggle against old age are not fitting goals for individuals in their own lives or for a health care system.

For all of the good that health represents, there are some important points to keep in mind as it is sought. The most important of these is that **there is no perfect correlation between health and happiness, betwen length of life and satisfaction with life, or between the health of individuals and their common good as a community.** Good health can help us live better lives, but the final meaning and value of life will not ordinarily turn on the state of our health. More important will be that we make of the living of a life of which health is the means. A recognition of limits can be understood to encompass the acceptance of a full (but not necessarily biologically maximum) life span, death from conditions whose eradication would require an unreasonable expenditure of resources, and a circumscribed place for the pursuit of health as a societal good.

We have now reached that point in medical and health history where an acceptance of limits requires that some important frontiers be restricted, and strong fences with small gates built at those frontiers. This is the only way to make clear to ourselves that we are prepared to live within limits, and the only way in practice that we can <u>ever</u> hope to manage our healthcare resources in some sensible fashion. There are two frontiers that must be restricted. One of these is along the temporal axis of aging, the other along the curative axis of individual need. The most imperative first step in the institution of restrictions is to acknowledge that both frontiers are open and endless, never to be conquered. They admit of no known natural, self-limiting boundaries, though some have been speculated upon.

A. <u>The Frontier of Aging</u>: Most of us now alive will die beyond the age of 65. That means that the future of medical progress, at least in terms of dealing with the highest proportion of mortality, lies with the cure or amelioration of conditions afflicting the elderly. There is no dream so powerful for many than that of wholly separating becoming sick and becoming old, of making old age a wholly new, improved state of life, "the beginning of a new life" as one popular slogan in the United States has it. The hope is what might be called the modernization of aging. Yet we should know that this is an illusion, even if we can make some substantial progress. No matter what progress is made with the unwanted conditions of old age - sickness, disability, the fading of youthful powers - there will always be others to take their place. The body will insist upon decline and decay, later if not sooner, but always implacably. The cure of one disease or condition will always be followed by another condition requiring cure, and then another, and then another, and so on indefinitely.

While it will no doubt be impossible and undesirable to wholly restrict efforts to extend life at that frontier of aging, we can ask a special question of the social health care system: what is a reasonable length of life to which people can aspire and which we might together seek to attain? I believe that, if we could get most people through a typically full biographical life-span, by which I mean the late 70s or early 80s, we will have done them a decent service. By that time most people will have had the opportunity to raise a family, to work, to love, to travel, to enjoy, to make of themselves what they want to be. For many that task will never be completed, and for others it will be completed much sooner. For the system as a whole, however, we can aim for a common general level, and certainly most people will have done what can be done by the early 80s.

While it is true of course that notions of a decent biographical life span will be different to some extent for different people, it cannot be the obligation of the health care system to orient itself to a kind of curative medicine that is hostage to individual life plans and desires beyond a reasonably full life span. That should always be understood as optional on its part. I can understand why someone would want to live to 105, but it is not evident I am required, as his fellow citizen and fellow human being, to contribute support toward helping him achieve through expensive medical means that highly individualized goal. I should have helped him with preventive medicine early in his life, with immunization as a child, and with decent primary care, but I am not required to help him pursue unlimited life. We are not required to follow the culture of modernized aging wherever it might lead, especially when we come to know what it will cost, and how little in improved happiness we might get anyway. A society would, then, be well justified in the future to set an age limit on the public provision of expensive, life-extending, curative health care (though always required to provide the kind of caring outlined above).

B. *Frontier of Individual Cure*: The second limit is on individual cure. If the possibilities of extending life through time are unending (an ever-increasing average life expectancy and a drawing out of old age), so also are the possibilities of effecting the cure of individuals of all ages. Here we encounter the phenomenon of what might be called the vertical gap which shows it increasingly possible to spend ever-larger amounts of money to save the lives of desperately ill individuals (in the United States 1.5-2 million dollar cases). This growing phenomenon makes clear that, however far we go with medical progress for the individual, we can never find a place to tear the cloth of progress that does not leave a ragged edge, that edge which represents the limits of our present knowledge and skills, ever-transcendable, never-conquerable. That is a frontier we cannot best, and which needs to be restricted also - not necessarily closed altogether, but closed in the sense that we work to erect a strong fence around it, one that has openings for progress, but small, restrictive ones, subject to powerful restraints.

Yet the problem of restricting this frontier is more difficult in principle than restricting the frontier of aging. It is evident that any attempt to do so would be seen as a challenge to a key feature of our entire Western way of life, our belief in the unlimited pursuit of progress. It is also harder to imagine finding a place to draw a line on the provision of curative medicine for individuals than to find a place to draw a line on curative health care and life extension for the elderly as a group. In the case of aging at least, there are cultural traditions of what counts as a "full" life, even if the borders are hazy. All efforts to find good individual standards, by contrast, have fared poorly. However well-devised, notions of cost-effective care, or standards based on "quality of life", or norms of acceptable outcome, are not likely to work well for individual cure. They will run aground on different beliefs of what counts as a benefit, or a decent quality of life, beliefs made problematic precisely because of a constant medical progress able to draw out some benefit, some quality, even in the most severe illnesses.

We must, then approach this frontier differently than can be possible with aging. Yet we must do so with a willingness, seen before we set out, to understand that it is a restriction we are about, that one way or another we must abandon the idea of unlimited progress on the frontier of individual curative need. The question is not whether, but where and how. For that we need a set, first, of aspirations and then, second, priorities within those aspirations; and then some quidelines on the management of technology.

2. Making Decisions: Categorical or Individual?

When we have to set limits, or establish treatment standards, is that best done on an individual, case-by-case, basis, or by the use of what I will call categorical standards? In general, I believe, it will become increasingly necessary to move a long way toward categorical standards and to firm protocols for treatment. The most common norm at present is that of individual physician judgment, usually but not always in consultation with patients and their families. These judgments are ordinarily based on loose, often tacit professional standards and practices, and often as well on the personal standards of physicians. By a categorical standard I mean, in contrast, the use of some relatively objective, required, public standards for the provision of particular forms of healthcare, or for the cessation or limiting of care. Examples would be the use of age as a limit on some forms of treatment for the elderly, and the use of firm outcome or other efficacy standards for other patients. Such standards may be that, say, of a minimal weight limit for premature newborns as a condition for aggressive efforts to preserve the life of the baby (as in Sweden); firm, objective criteria for admission to intensive care units (as is now the case in many American hospitals, but implemented in too loose a fashion); the relative likelihood of significant benefit based on some objective standard from a treatment; or the elimination of some expensive forms of therapy altogether, whatever their benefit, on grounds of cost or relatively poor long-term outcomes.

I recognize that a movement toward categorical standards will raise serious problems concerning traditional medical values. The attraction of individual decisions by individual physicians - will this patient benefit from this treatment? - is that they seem most to respect our differences as persons, both in what we want and in our physical condition. They are, in that respect, consistent with moral traditions of medicine, oriented as they are to individual patient welfare and considerable physician discretion. They are among our most cherished values.

How can I possibly argue that such deep and revered standards may have to be set aside or modified in many circumstances? There are three reasons. The first is that, in the face of the limitless possibilities of cure, it will utterly be out of the question for a society to do everything that might benefit individual patients; it is the demand for maximum individual choice and benefit that is iself a powerful source of our problem. Is there an alternative? Yes. If a limit must be set, it will be much less of an assault upon individual dignity to deny a patient curative, beneficial care because it is _this_ patient. It would be the relative efficacy of a treatment, or its availability to a particular group - based upon publicly announced and openly visible standards - that would determine treatment reimbursement, not subjective physician, patient, or family judgments about relative patient worth or quality of life. Individuals can be brought to understand and accept that society might not be able to give them all they want or need. But that will be possible only if it is done in a way that shows they are not being singled out for special discrimination, because of who they are personally, and only if they believe that the general good of society is thereby being served. They must, of course, always have the assurance that, if they cannot have all the curative medicine they might want, they will never be abandoned. They will always receive basic care for the relief of pain and suffering - categorical limits would be used only to set limits to curative medicine, not to the provision of care and caring.

The second reason is that it is simply impossible to carry out large-scale rationing and limitation policies at the bedside. We know from well over two decades of trying how hard it is to make termination decisions with individual patients even when the desire is simply to serve the welfare of the patient and resource allocation is not a consideration. Physicians differ among themselves, family members disagree, and sometimes doctors and patients cannot agree. The important moral tradition that always gives the benefit of doubt to treatment, and the no less potent tradition of medical ethics which does exactly the same, together work to make it exceedingly difficult to stop treatment or deny any possibly beneficial procedures or tests, so much so that overtreatment or unwanted treatment may be common. If asked, then, to carry out rationing policies at the bedside, those traditions would not only put physicians in the unsavory and painful position of having to personally execute policies of limits and rationing with their individual patients, but there is also every likelihood that it would not work in any case. It would invite both evasion of general standards, or the application of personal, perhaps capricious standards, unfair and insensitive in many cases. Categorical standards, imposed from the outside and setting limits to the actions of physicians in a decisive way would avoid those problems. The goal would be not so much to tell physicians in oppressive detail what they must do in treating patients, as to establish standards of what would not be acceptable at the outer boundaries. It would be imperative that physicians have a central role in helping to set such standards. They must be compatible with physician integrity, and that integrity need not entail a claim that every patient has a maximum claim on maximum resources whatever to societal costs.

The third reason is that categorical standards are open to inspection, subject to debate, clean and clear in their application. That is why they have proved attractive in many other public policy contexts, where an individualized approach would not work well: the setting of a minimal age to drive, or to drink, or to serve in the armed forces; the use of a specific speed limit on highways; and the use of hard standards on vision and hearing for, say, airline pilots and drivers. Inevitably, categorical standards are unfair to individuals; we are different as individuals. But the overall balance of fairness and policy clarity can make categorical standards valuable for public programs.

In arguing for the need for limits, I do so in order that we might be forced to keep before our eyes, and imbedded in our policies, some powerful and enduring tensions. I have in mind the tension between our acceptance of finitude and our aspiration for boundless progress; between our individual needs and desires and the needs of the common good; between our quest for health as a human good and the necessity to commit resources to other societal goods. By our now deeply ingrained modern belief in unlimited medical progress, we have falsely persuaded ourselves that we can have it all, that we can do away with the tensions. We can not. No less importantly, in order to set meaningful medical priorities, we must work within a set of limits. Otherwise we will never take seriously the idea of priorities at all. We will delude ourselves into thinking that greater efficiency, or more research, will obviate the need for priorities. A lively sense of limits, by contrast, will underline the necessity for priorities. To accept them is nothing other than to understand that, while we can have much that we dream of in the name of improved health, we can not have everything.

Ethics in Medicine, edited by
Peter Allebeck and Bengt Jansson.
Raven Press, New York © 1990.

PRIORITIES FOR TREATMENT WITH HIGHLY SPECIALIZED TECHNOLOGY – BONE MARROW TRANSPLANTATION

Gösta Gahrton

Bone marrow transplantation is a relatively new method to treat patients with a variety of disorders. The most common indication for bone marrow transplantation is leukemia, but non-malignant disorders such as aplastic anemia and genetic diseases are also important indications. There are two types of bone marrow transplantation, i.e. allogeneic bone marrow transplantation and autologous bone marrow transplantation.

Allogeneic transplantation involves the transfer of bone marrow from a donor which is usually a sibling, but can also be an unrelated donor who is matched immunologically for the HLA (human leukocyte antigen) locus. Allogeneic bone marrow transplantation can be used for treatment of patients with leukemia. Technically, allogeneic bone marrow transplantation involves pretreatment (conditioning), infusion of bone marrow, and graft-versus-host-disease prevention after the infusion of marrow. The conditioning treatment eradicates the marrow by supralethal cytotoxic drug therapy, total body irradiation or both. The patient is thereafter rescued by the infusion of the normal bone marrow from the donor. In neoplastic disorders, the conditioning treatment is used for two purposes, i.e. firstly for killing neoplastic cells and secondly for eradicating immunologically active cells that could reject the transplant. The price for the curative treatment is that normal cells are also killed. Therefore, the patient needs to be rescued by the allogeneic marrow. In other conditions, such as aplastic anemia or the genetic disorders, the conditioning treatment is solely used to prevent rejection of the graft.

In autologous bone marrow transplantation, the patient is his/hers own donor. The marrow is collected from the patients, frozen and stored during the conditioning period. The conditioning is used to kill malignant cells, for example in leukemia. The marrow is then reinfused in the patient in order to save him or her from the supralethal conditioning therapy.

Bone marrow transplantation requires special resources, such as highly specialized personnel, reversed insolation units, expensive cytotoxic drugs and antibiotics, and total body irradiation. The

Figure 1   **PRIORITIZING FOR BONE MARROW TRANSPLANTATION**

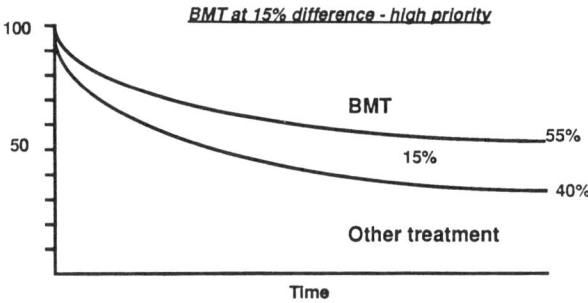

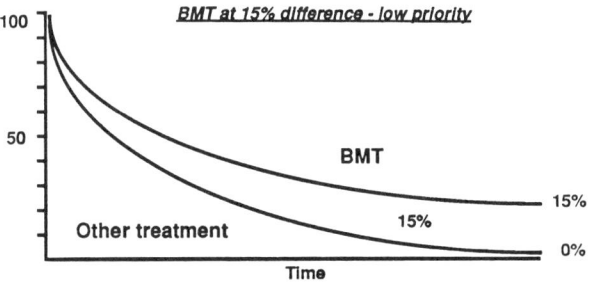

Table 1

Prioritizing for allogeneic bone marrow transplantation in acute lymphoblastic leukemia..

Diagnosis	Stage	Expected survival		Priority
		Other methods	BMT	
ALL, children standard risk	1st CR	60-70%	60-70%	None
ALL, children high risk	1st CR	30-40%	50-60%	High
ALL, children	2nd CR	5-15%	25-35%	Very high
ALL, adults <50 years	1st CR	20-40%	45-50%	High
ALL, adults <50 years	2nd CR	0-5%	20-30%	Very high
ALL	Relapse	0	5-20%	Low-none

immediate cost for bone marrow transplantation is high, around U.S. dollar 100,000. It involves the investment in localities, machinery, and personnel, Thus, although it is not more costly than chemotherapy when calculated as the cost per saved year of life, most countries have limited resources for investment in this highly specialized technology. Prioritizing is therefore a continuous problem and takes into account several aspects, i.e. medical, health-care-personnel-related, and resource-related ones. Firstly, bone marrow transplantation is only used if it gives a better chance to cure than other treatment modalities, such as conventional chemotherapy. If the chances to cure are similar, the judgement does not involve difficulties because immediate transplant-related complications are more severe than immediate complications with chemotherapy. Bone marrow transplantation is therefore no choice, and chemotherapy is used instead. On the other hand, if bone marrow transplantation is superior, but not dramatically so, the decision is difficult. Other factors than pure medical ones are therefore considered, i.e. the magnitude of the fraction of patients cured with bone marrow transplantation, the limitation of resources and the capacity of the health care personnel to cope with the complications of bone marrow transplantation. An example of outcome of the decision in acute lymphoblastic leukemia is seen in Table 1 and Figure 1. If there is about a 15-percent difference in bone marrow transplantation and other treatment it is performed only in those categories of patients who have a relatively high success rate (>15% cured) with the methodology but not in those with a low (<15% cured) predicted success rate, although none in this group can be cured without bone marrow transplantation. This kind of prioritizing can be debated but appears to be the only possible one if resources are limited and if the psychological capacity of the personnel should be maintained. Increased resources and intensive psychological back-up of the team might help in changing the priorities in order to treat the poor prognostic category of patients. However, in most transplant centers a 15-20 percent success rate appears to be a required limit.

In summary, setting priorities for bone marrow transplantation is a difficult task and many factors, not only medical ones, are involved in the decision-making process.

Ethics in Medicine, edited by
Peter Allebeck and Bengt Jansson.
Raven Press, New York © 1990.

PRIORITIES FOR ADVANCED TECHNOLOGY IN THE DIAGNOSIS AND TREATMENT OF PATIENTS WITH HEART DISORDERS

Olof Edhag

About half of the death rate in Western countries is related to cardiovascular diseases, which means that there are enormous demands for medical care in this field, both from patients suffering from heart disease and from the community as a whole for example in the form of preventive measures.

As in other medical fields, the progress in cardiology has accelerated dramatically since the beginning of this century. When Eindhoven invented the electrocardiograph in 1903 the enormous importance of this apparatus could not be foreseen. The development of electrocardiography has been one of the principal milestones in cardiological innovations.

Although Adams-Stokes' syndrome - brief attacks of cardiac standstill with syncopal episodes due to heart block - was described as early as in the 17th century, it was not until the 1950s, when transistors and capacitors became available, that this condition could be treated and began to be systematically searched for. The Swedish company which in 1958 constructed the first implantable pacemaker in the world asked some experienced cardiologists in Sweden about the need for this device in this country. The number of bradyarrhythmias that were treatable by artificial heart stimulation was at that time calculated to be about 50 in the whole country. Today almost 2.000 Swedes - 40 times more than was anticipated - are supplied with new pacemaker systems annually. It is thus difficult to predict the need for a method, an apparatus or a device when it is first introduced.

Problems related to indications for pacing today mostly concern the question of what system will be optimal for a particular patient. We now have access to more sophisticated and of course also more expensive systems than three decades ago. It has to be considered what diagnostic procedures should be carried out before it is decided to implant a pacemaker and before the mode of stimulation is selected. Another matter of importance concerning pacemaker treatment is to what extent the devices can be re-used. In some pacemaker centres in Sweden hundreds of thousands of Swedish kronor are saved every year by re-using pacemakers. In others, not a single generator is re-used. In the United States legal aspects, if I am correctly informed, have made it impossible to re-use pacemakers. To what extent is the doctor able to make decisions in this matter? Is it a question for the county councils that have to defray the costs or for the National Board of Health and Welfare, which is reponsible for seeing that an adequate level of health care is provided in the country? What are the reasons for the differences between countries? Hardly biological - but possible legal or economic?

Another question concerning the resources is how far we should go in our search for untreated diseases and undetected disorders in the community. The more we search for, the more we find. This case illustrates this question.

A 56-year-old apparently healthy athletic man was reported on by Marmor & Black (1). He appeared to have a sinus bradycardia with a heart rate of 30/minute during the daytime and as low as 11/minute when asleep. He was furnished with a pacemaker. To what extent should we as specialists be involved in screening of the population for treatable conditions? In Sweden we specialists are responsible for health care, not only at our own department but also in the catchment area outside the hospitals.

In patients with arrhythmias it is possible today to reveal the mechanism underlying a specific arrhythmia by recording of an intracardiac electrogram combined with a stimulation technique. With this method an arrhythmia may also be induced and terminated. In this way different antiarrhythmic drugs may be tested. Some of these arrhythmias are life-threatening. This technique is used today in three centers in Sweden, which means that for a patient, the question of whether your arrhythmia is properly investigated or not depends quite a lot on where you live and how informed your general practitioner is. If drugs are not effective as treatment of some severe potentially life-threatening arrhythmias, it is possible today to implant an automatic defibrillator which will deliver an electric shock and terminate ventricular tachyarrhythmias. In Stockholm one such unit has hitherto been implanted and in all of Sweden, five. In just one hospital in New York, 150 have been implanted. The cost of every unit is about 20.000 US dollars. There are several reasons for not implanting such devices in our hospital, although we have the ability both to perform the investigations required and to implant the units. One reason is that there is no money in the budget for this treatment. Another, more important, reason than budget restrictions is lack of knowledge among patients and general practitioners that this treatment is available today. What are our responsibilities as specialists to inform the general practitioners and the public about new techniques?

The availability of safe and well-functioning equipment is of great importance in modern medicine and not least in cardiology. A 36-year-old man, previously healthy, attended the Emergency Department of the hospital for chest pain. ECG revealed unspecific changes. Echocardiography showed severe dilated cardiomyopathy, a disease which is treated with drugs with several side effects and not seldom has a poor prognosis. However, at a second investigation with another equipment, the findings were absolutely normal; the patient was in fact healthy. Thus, unreliable equipments might cause harm to the patient and create unnecessary costs.

For optimal fulfilment of his or her tasks, the cardiologist needs expensive equipment, implantable devices, and sleight of hand to be able to manipulate catheters properly. Not least, knowledge and experience are of great importance for adequate treatment. For the cardiac surgeon operative skill is mandatory.

In one respect the cardiologist holds a special position in the medical family, in that he or she carries out invasive cardiac procedures many of which are potentially dangerous for the patient if the cardiologist is not sufficiently well-trained or if he is not adequately supervised during training. The first principle of human behaviour - to help and never hurt - is obvious for all doctors in their professional work. But when performing angiography and angioplastic procedures the cardiologist cannot promise there will be no risk to the patient. In cardiology this basic principle is thus relative. Angioplasty is a technique whereby narrowed coronary vessels can be opened up. Complications such as acute myocardial infarction occur in about 5 per cent and ventricular fibrillation, a life-threatening arrhythmia, in about one per cent. Furthermore, angiographically verifiable re-stenosis can occur in 30-35 per cent within a reasonable length of time (2). The cardiologist performing the procedure must, of course, be aware of the absolute contraindications. It has also been shown that some categories of patients are more favourable regarding the chances of success, such as those below 65 years of age, male patients, and patients with single-vessel disease. The patient must, of course, be informed about the risk in relation to the benefit before the procedure. He or she must also be told about the success rate and the percentage of re-stenosis. This example illustrates the importance of adequate training and supervision of invasive cardiologists. It should be stated that it is unethical to expose patients to unnecessary investigations and treatments by reason of insufficient traing on the part of the physician or defective equipment. The American College of Cardiology has formulated guidelines for cardiologists performing different invasive procedures (2).

Another question which should be considered in the discussion on invasive procedures, is how to handle patients who are HIV-positive. Doctors of course have no right to refuse to investigate a patient for such a reason. A doctor's knowledge does not belong to him or her alone but to the community.

An important question is to what extent the doctor, being responsible for the resources, has the right to have one patient operated on before another. This case report illustrates one aspect of this dilemma:

A 33-year-old man was referred to Huddinge Hospital because of angina pectoris. He was a Polish immigrant. He had had hypertension since the age of 18 years and also had diabetes. He was a heavy smoker and was overweight (20%).

When he came to us he was getting angina after walking on level ground for only 30-100 meters, in spite of "optimal medication". ECG showed an old diaphragmal myocardial infaction. Coronary angiography revealed advanced atherosclerosis with five sites of narrowing, which was considered treatable by bypass surgery.

There has been a deficiency of resources both for coronary angiography and for bypass surgery in Sweden during the last decade.

Should the risk factors of these patients (smoking, over-weight, hypercholesterolaemia) be corrected before they are accepted for bypass surgery?

To what extent and how vigorously is it justifiable for a physician to try to change the patient's habits and should he refuse treatment until the lifestyle has been changed?

A very destructive debate on technology in medical care took place at the beginning of 1970s. Ivan Illich wrote in 1975 (3):

> "The harm of medical care is an epidemic spreading more rapidly than most others. Diseases caused by doctors have an influence on costs for health care exceeding those of traffic accidents or war".

We who are responsible for highly specialized care, and of course the patients in need of our resources, still suffer from these discussions when we argue in favour of new equipment.

On the other hand, with the increasing costs for both investigations and medical treatment, the question should be raised if it is justified for any doctor to order any investigation and prescribe any treatment.

In all Western countries it is obvious that today we have possibilities, to an extent never experienced before, of diagnosing and treating symptoms and also of finding symptom-free disorders that are correctable. The demand for health care seems to be unlimited. Treatments differ considerably not only between countries but also within a country. If you are a patient, select the country when you need health care, and also the city. Find out how well-informed your general practitioner is. Also, try to find out how well trained your specialist is, if you happen to know the one you will need.

There have been attempts to compare different forms of treatment in the cardiological field concerning cost-benefit and cost-efficacy - also taking into account quality of life. Even if this kind of comparison is relevant, who is to make the decisions after the analysis have been performed? The discussion about how to make priorities must be intensified. Doctors/politicians/administrators have hitherto only touched upon the question of how to solve the enormous priority problems with which we are now faced. These problems will certainly increase during the next decade. We need probably expertise outside the medical community to find systems for sharing the resources for medical care in as optimal a way as possible.

To conclude, the following points raised illustrate the type of ethical issues that are involved in clinical decision making in cardiology.

1) It is difficult to predict the need for a new method when it is first introduced. From this it follows, that when a new method becomes available, those who will benefit from it will be found more by chance than after systematic analyses. How active should we be in our search for untreated diseases or undetected disorders in the community?

2) To what extent should we inform colleagues outside our speciality and the public (community) about new expensive methods which have proved to be, or show indications of being beneficial?

3) How high a degree of sohpistication should we

allow or strive for when so many are in need of the resources?

4) Some investigations in cardiology are potentially dangerous. The university and the hospital (county council) are responsible for adequate training of those who are to perform advanced procedures.

5) The hospital is responsible for exchange of defective equipment.

6) Is it ever justified to refuse treatment because the patient's life-style is destructive?

7) Can we refuse to treat patients with diseases that are potentially dangerous to the medical staff? (In my opinion no).

8) How far do our responsibilities go as clinicians in making priorities among our own patients or patient categories?

References

1. Marmor, B.M., Black, M.M.: Unusual manifestations of severe sick sinus syndrome. Am Heart J 1980; 100:95-98.

2. ACC/AHA Task force report: Guidelines for percutaneous transluminal coronary angioplasty. A report of the American College of Cardiology and Therapeutic Cardiovascular Procedures. JACC 1988; 12:529-45.

3. Illich, I.: Quoted in Ord och Bild 1975:84 no 6 (in Swedish).

RATIONING AND PRIORITY SETTING: DISCUSSION

Shimon Glick

I should like to begin by expressing my sense of discomfort and uneasiness that most of the erudite discussions about rationing health care resources and allocating priorities take place in some on the wealthiest societies in human history, while simultaneously in many of the underdeveloped areas of the world, people are dying every minute of poverty, starvation and preventable illness. The decisions in those countries are made without symposia, by Darwinian survival of the fittest in all its stark cruelty. In parts of Africa, if a mother gives birth to twins, only one is brought to her, because she lacks milk to feed two. In our societies that discuss "tragic choices" in health care, one trillion dollars are spent annually, almost three billion dollars daily, on military expenditures. I believe these sobering contrasts should not be forgotten in our deliberations when we discuss "lack of resources". It seems to me that were we, as a collective human endeavor, being observed from another planet, the observers would surely judge our collective self-destructive and mutually destructive behavior as incontrovertible evidence of mass insanity.

Having forgotten that statement off my chest, I will try to address some of the issues raised by the previous speakers and by the subject at hand.

In a 1984 New England Journal of Medicine article (1), Victor Fuchs referred to a statement that "the United States will soon have to begin rationing medical care" as "sheer nonsense", because rationing and setting of priorities both on a micro and a macro level have been with us since the dawn of time. They are inevitable and ubiquitous phenomena, whether overt or undiagnosed. Resources, by their nature, are finite, whereas perceived or real needs of society are virtually infinite. There are folk proverbs in many cultures which describe man's insatiable appetite in _every_ sphere, not just in health. While the magnitude and quality of the gap between needs and resources vary strikingly from society to society, with some countries spending several hundred times more per capita on health care than others, all societies have huge and growing gaps. The realities of modern medicine, with its almost unparallelled capabilities and its potentially almost infinite and growing costs, relentlessly confront those who would deny the necessity for painful decisions.

The first step in the process of setting health care priorities is the frank admission that even the wealthiest societies cannot provide unlimited services for all, and that all societies, and all physicians, consciously or unwittingly, are constantly setting priorities. In view of the unavoidability of priority setting, it would therefore seem preferable to examine our actions prospectively, in a rational and critical manner. The individual physician rations the time and energy he devotes to each patient. He decides whom to see first and for how long, which problem to defer and which to treat. He does not sit with his patient around the clock, and most reasonable patients accept this form of rationing. Every society sets priorities. Government budgets decide how much will go to health in its narrow sense, how much will go to other needs such as education, housing, highways and similar areas which influence health and how much to functions that may actually be detrimental to health. Then, there are the decisions within the officially designated health budgets as to where the limited resources go, preventive versus therapeutic, young versus old, rehabilitation versus emergency and the like. Decisions, decisions, all the time.

The myriad decisions make those of legendary King Solomon seem easy. I think even he would have had trouble coping with today's complex choices. It is encouraging that in the spirit of glasnost, we are talking about the problems more openly, debating them, and analysing them from philosophical, ethical, economic and medical points of view. But in trying to solve our problems rationally, it is important that we avoid self deception. We have finally succeeded in shattering the illusion that we can and do give every patient the maximum possible. Most of us are now aware as individuals and societies that we are limited and finite. But it is essential that in man's infinite capacity for self delusion and rationalization, we do not replace the old delusions with new ones. I hope none of us believes that these problems are soluble to everyones satisfaction or that the answer can be found to the problem in priority setting. I suggest too that we do not deceive ourselves by exaggerating the magnitude of the problem and its temporal uniqueness and urgency, so that we do not plunge panic stricken into unwise and immoral solutions.

Many thoughtful individuals are still haunted by memories of the ethical horrors which resulted in the past from purely utilitarian decisions. Our Western religious cultural antecedents have, at least in theory, emphasized protection of the weak, often at great cost. All too many countries unfortunately remain plagued by the existence of substantial, unjustified disparities in the availability of health care between the different strata of society. Given the tendency of groups to be concerned most with their own welfare, and given the potential "tyranny" of the majority in democratic societies and the overt tyranny of the ruling classes in totalitarian regimes, a real danger exists that weaker segments of society may easily be shortchanged with regard to health care resources. I hope that somehow we have made progress over the millenia and need not revert to solutions which characterized the Spartan society's coping with limited resources. It would also be sad indeed, if the richest societies in human history would resort to solutions similar to those that are being tragically imposed daily in impoverished Africa and Asia. I believe we can and must do better.

There is no single formula for how to set either macro or micro priorities. Without meaning to deprecate Raanan Gillon's erudite philosophic discussion as to the different theories of medical resource allocation, I must admit that I enjoyed even more Raanan's description in the British Medical Journal (2) of his eight year old daughter's analysis of how to choose one of three dying patients for the only lifesaving dialysis machine. Her quoted list of options and choices was very close to that of much more professional philosophers who merely expressed the options in more conventional professional jargon. But I will not attempt here to improve on either Raanan's or his daugter's analysis.

Each society will have to struggle within its particular value system and within its own fiscal and organizational constraints, to reach solutions which are perceived to be equitable by its citizens, and which can stand up to critical scrutiny by "objective" standards of justice and fairness. The process of setting the necessary criteria should involve individuals and groups from a variety of disciplines, should be sensitive to the potential prejudices and biases of these decision makers, and should be subject to continued critical evaluation and revision in accord with new data and insights.

I do, however, wish to take strong issue with Dan Callahan's well articulated and by now well publicized position on setting categorical age limits for curative therapy (3, 4). I think this view is misguided and wrong, medically, ethically and perhaps even economically. Firstly, the issue is presented in a way which I am not sure is correct. It is alleged that the problem of the expensive care for the elderly lies largely in the high technology acute care, the curative phase. The implication is that were we to change the orientation from curing or healing to caring or helping, we could save money. I question that simplistic postulate, which sets up technology as some devil reincarnated, the source of all evil. Long term decent caring kind of help may actually be equally expensive or even more so, requiring enormous quantities of personal nursing care over a very long period. And if we take that route, the same questions that are now being asked about expensive curative therapy wil soon be focussed on the high cost of caring. My guess is that a similar answer will emerge - that is, an arbitrary limitation of care. In fact, Margaret Battin in a recent book entitled "Should Medical Care be Rationed by Age" (5) suggests encouraging, or at least permitting voluntary suicide. The reasons cited are that with rationing imposed on the elderly, palliative care too will be rationed, making the quality of life unbearable. The argument states that we were to create a social morality encouraging suicide, there might be enough people taking advantage of that option that the need for hard rationing might be alleviated. In a review of her position (6), Paul Menzel suggests that linking of rationing of palliative care and permission of suicide, in his words "seems premature". But "premature" events often do eventually occur - sooner than expected. Dan Callahan cites the five fold rise in Mayo Clinic surgery performed on those over 90 - which sounds dramatic and impressive. I venture though that the absolute numbers were trivial in terms of their contribution to the overall costs of the Mayo Clinic, and that the outcomes were quite impressive as well.

Furthermore, I am not convinced that removing the 80 year old from the intensive care unit will save all that much money, simply because intensive care unit beds are rarely left open. The 80 year old will usually be replaced with a 20 or a 60 year old with the actual net savings far less than promised.

I frankly am disturbed at the full implications of the Callahan approach if followed precisely as outlined. According to this approach, if we have a patient over our agreed age limit who is in coma with meningitis, he should not receive antibiotics. He is not suffering, and the treatment is just to prolong life - which has now been ruled inappropriate for this age. This is a shocking conclusion which few physicans could or should accept. One frequently encounters the reflex rejection of advanced technology for older people especially by non-physicians. Yet, by so doing, one may actually create greater morbidity and cost. Take implantation of a cardiac pacemaker in an 85 year old man with frequent fainting attacks. The pacemaker may prevent that man from being homebound, may prevent a hip fracture with its attendant hospitalization, disability and expense. Hip nailing in a 90 year old woman is cheaper than permitting her to remain bedridden for months or years. Expensive technology is often cheaper than the alternative.

Dr. Callahan makes it clear that his proposal requires categorical rules and cannot work if left to individual discretion and that we, as a society, should decide at what age its members have lived their full lives and have enjoyed, or perhaps suffered, a reasonable array of life experiences. Just a few weeks ago, I spent an afternoon with a 92 year old professor of history of medicine who is still an alert scholar, full of the desire and ability to contribute in his field, and very active in the guidance of young scholars who find him a most unusual and fertile resource. In fact, last week, he returned to me a superbly edited and critiqued work of one of our graduate students in the history of medicine. I remember visiting him in the hospital just a few years earlier after an accident. In that hospital setting, traumatized by the accident, febrile and confused, he was just a doddering old man, barely able to cope with his basic bodily functions - certainly not deserving of hospital care to prolong his life. I remember those very thoughts crossing my mind then. Yet, he has had, and still has, years in which he has contributed significantly to society and to his family - in fact, more so than many, many younger citizens.

I simply cannot accept any arbitrary and categorical cut-off by any outsider as to when as individual has accomplished his reasonable life goals - and paradoxically, this proposal emerges from a society that has made personal autonomy almost its highest ethical priority. This approach violates the principles of autonomy and integrity which were discussed so eloquently this morning.

Saddest of all, in my opinion, is that an insufficient attempt has been made to examine critically and comprehensively, the cause and magnitude of the problems with the elderly and to seek solutions other than to limit therapy for them. The longer life of individuals in our society is only a small facet of the problem. Since a good portion of the added years is composed of healthy active years, much of problem is due perhaps more to earlier retirement, shorter work week, a reduced birth rate and other factors that have reduced the productive work years of the population that has to foot the bill. A reduction of physician's fees, drug and insurance company profits and other possible cost excesses might be more fruitful foci for reducing health care costs than an arbitrary age cut off for the elderly. I am confident that there are more imaginative, intelligent and humane solutions to the health problems of the elderly.

One of the principal foundations with which medical education has endeavored to imbue students is the individuality of each patient. We teach that a careful physician takes into account every source of data, biological, physiological and sociocultural, before raching a therapeutic decision. We emphasize that there are 45 year olds who are physiologically older than 70 year olds and vice versa. I believe that only a non physician could propose an arbitrary boundary for treatment by chronological age. If such a demarcation were accepted, it would damage seriously the scientific, as well as the holistic, approach to the patient, and would contradict the basic principles of sound medicine which educators have labored long and hard to inculcate.

The Callahan plan has a number of serious defects from an ethical point of view as well. Albert Einstein once proposed as a criterion for a humane and civilized society, the way they treat their elderly. The relegating of the aged to the medical discard heap is a very serious step, with grave ethical implications. The elderly already have been singularly discriminated against in modern Western societies, which are youth and achievement oriented, and the aged represent an easy mark for further victimization - although I must admit that with their increasing numbers and political clout, they are reversing this trend remarkably and effectively.

The categorical age guideline also is simply bad medicine, with detrimental impact on the way the physician approaches and deals with the individual patient and his needs. The aged have long expressed justifiable dissatisfaction with physicians, and they have charged that their complaints are treated far too casually and condescendingly by physicians, with disparaging remarks such as "Well what do you expect at your age". When a patient, complaining of pain in his right knee, was given this offhand reply by his physician, he appropriately replied "But Doc, the left knee is just as old as the right, but it doesn't hurt". Age alone is not the answer.

The proposed automatic cut off may aggravate communication barriers between patients and their physicians and give an official stamp of approval for the confirmation of another group of second class citizens. This attitude must inevitably erode the fabric of medicine in its classic role of making a maximal effort for every patient to save life _and_ relieve suffering, in accord with the <u>specific</u> needs and desires of the patient, using the physician's best professional judgement. This approach would also impair the trust between patients and their physicians, described so eloquently in the paper by Dr. Pellegrino.

The adoption of an arbitrary age deadline gives us two equally unpalatable alternatives for those elderly who insist on curative and expensive therapy. One can permit such therapy only for those who have the means, not an attractive option. The other possibility, that of forbidding such expenditure even for the wealthy, is equally unacceptable in most democratic societies.

Does this mean that we must treat every elderly person maximally with every possible expensive therapy, and that we must thereby cause unnecessary and unwanted suffering? Medical priority decisions are made daily and the data are clear everywhere that the elderly <u>are</u> given far less of the high tech, dangerous and difficult therapies than are young people (7). But this is an individual decision, based hopefully on comprehensive evaluation of the patient as a whole, his or her desires and aspirations, the potential benefits from the treatment and the dangers and discomforts - just as we evaluate every other patient. This limitation of therapy in many older patients for medical reasons is quite natural and appropriate since with increasing age, risks increase, and benefits decrease. Therefore, many procedures are performed less commonly on the elderly. But tragically, data indicate that for identical benefit/cost ratios, the elderly are <u>already</u> discriminated against and deprived of standard acceptable care. This was shown recently (8) in a study of breast cancer therapy in patients with a potential for cure, where patients matched for severity of illness and life expectancy, were clearly shortchanged if over 70 years of age. Official sanction of such discrimination would only worsen an already unfortunate and unjustified reality.

One often hears the argument that rather than spend more on curative treatment for the elderly, we should give better chronic nursing home care and the like. The clear implication is that we can do either one or the other but not both, and that if we reduce expenditure in one area, funds will be diverted to the more desirable services. This earmarked diversion may be likely in a country with a fixed health budget system like Great Britain, but is far less inevitable in the kind of market economy that exists in the U.S. The money for curative medicine may very well be reduced but with little assurance that it will be directed as the proposal's proponents desire. More likely, the same economic pressures and the utilitarian view of the limited benefits in treating demented nursing home patients will prevent a major increase in chronic care as well, as I pointed out earlier.

Unfortunately, I believe that the proposals to limit care by specific age based criteria are not merely responses to urgent societal constraints, which do of course exist, but represent as well the result of an unequivocal change in societal values. Whereas only a short time ago, human life was regarded as having intrinsic sanctity, this societal value has been removed from the list of ethical priorities by many contemporary philosophers (9). Already in 1968 (10), Francis Crick was quoted in an editorial in Nature that from a biological point of view, "We cannot continue to regard all human life as sacred", and as a consequence, he suggested perhaps redefining death at perhaps 80 or 85 and birth at 2 days of age.

Callahan has not perhaps gone as far, but we are approaching that stage. There are already enormous pressures to change the current brain death definition, and Wikler (11), for instance, has proposed that in order to solve the problem how to deal with patients in a persistent vegetative state, we define that state as already dead. But almost simultaneously, the suggestion was made by Ezekiel Emanuel that patients with advanced Alzheimer's disease really are no different in any important way from those with the persistent vegetative state. Clearly, we seem to be heading down a dangerous and slippery road, and we cannot always be certain at what point the brakes will hold.

Less than two weeks ago, we marked the 50th anniversary of the German euthanasia program which resulted in the deaths of 70.000 Germans. In Alexander's classic analysis of the pathogenesis of the German physician's degradation (13), the major factor was judged to be a utilitarian set of values whereby the value of the individual was determined by his or her potential contribution to society.

Dependency and lack of productivity were devalued. Dr. Alexander already at that time reported what he felt were disturbing preliminary signs of similar tendencies in the United States. I hope we are not falling into that tragic trap.

I agree with Dr. Callahan that we do need categorical criteria to help us with guidelines for the limits to treatment. Categorical criteria and specific protocols, and the discussions that precede them, increase the likelihood of equity and rationality in distributing scarce resources and they provide guidance and support for individual physicians in reaching these difficult decisions. If these categorical criteria are arrived at by a process that provides an opportunity for participation by interested and knowledgeable groups and individuals and are logical and resonable, they can add immeasurably to the quality of medical care and of decision making. So I am all for such overt, explicit and rational measures. It is unfortunate that the need for rational setting of priorities has been set back by the unfortunate choice of age as a basis for withholding therapy. But with respect to all categorical protocols and guidelines, a word of caution is in order. Slavish adherence to protocols can at times be harmful. Justice should be tempered with mercy. There are and will have to be exceptions to all protocols, even if rationality is thereby impaired. As we know from experience, in all societies an identifiable patient or a grounded whale, or even a cat which falls into a well will evoke more sympathy and demand larger monetary expenditures than thousands of unidentified statistical lives. Logic and rationality do not always triumph, and perhaps they should not. After all, we are not computers but human beings with hearts and emotions, as well as minds.

In summary, rationing and priority setting are an inevitable feature of health care. Open, rational discussions are critical to the establishment of relatively objective and equitable processes of rationing and priority setting. I feel that protocols and categorical guidelines are valuable and should be established. But I regard categorical age guidelines as fraught with serious problems and fatally flawed. I would suggest that such guidelines be allowed to die quietly by withholding of life sustaining support, so that more rational and scientifically sound criteria can replace them.

References

1. Fuchs, V.R.: The "rationing" of medical care. N Eng J Med 1984;311:1572-1573.

2. Gillon, R.: Justice and allocation of medical resources. Br Med J 1985;291:266-268.

3. Callahan, D.: Terminating treatment: age as a standard. Hastings Center Report 1987;16:5 (October):21-25.

4. Callahan, D.: Setting limits: Medical goals in an aging society. N.Y. Simon and Schuster, 1987.

5. Smeeding, T.M. et al: Should medical care be relatively rationed by age. Totowa, M.J., Rowman and Littlefield, 1987.

6. Menzel, P.T.: Review essay. Bioethics 1989;3:245-253.

7. Gillick, M.: Limiting medical care: physicians' beliefs, physicians' behavior. J Am Ger Soc 1988;36:747-752.

8. Greenfield, S., Blanco, D., Elashoff, R. et al: Patterns of care related to age of breast cancer patients. JAMA 1987;257:2766-2770.

9. A report of the Hastings Institute. Guidelines on the termination of life-sustaining treatment and the care of the dying. 1987;Indiana Univ., Press, Bloomington, Indiana.

10. Editorial. Logic of biology. Nature (London) 1968;220, 429.

11. Wikler, D.: Not dead, not dying? Ethical categories and persistent vegetative state. Hastings Center Report 18:2 (February):41-47.

12. Emanuel, E.J.: Should physicians withhold life-sustaining care for patients who are terminally ill? Lancet 1988;I:106-108.

13. Alexander, L.: Medical science under dictatorship. N Eng J Med 1949;241:39-47.

Ethics in Medicine, edited by
Peter Allebeck and Bengt Jansson.
Raven Press, New York © 1990.

CLINICAL FREEDOM: WHERE ARE THE LIMITS TO THE FREEDOM OF DOCTORS?

Raymond Hoffenberg

I have not been able to trace the origins of the term Clinical Freedom but the concept was much in evidence in Britain in the debate that led up to the formation of the National Health Service (NHS). Nor have I been able to find a clear definition of the term; it appears to embrace the freedom of clinicians to make decisions about the care of their patients, independently and without interference. Essentially, it applies to freedom of judgement and action about the management of an individual patient, based on the assumed and accepted obligation of a doctor to regard the interests of his patient as paramount, to be set above all other interests. Doctors have other wider obligations to their professional bodies and to Society through which their clinical freedom, as defined above, might need to be constrained. For most matters, such constraints are accepted but there is an occasional conflict of interests that produces an awkward professional dilemma. In general, doctors defend their concept of clinical freedom vigorously and resist any change that might tend to diminish it.

In this paper I shall consider some changes that

have already taken place, which have reduced the clinician's freedom of action and which may do so more drastically in the future. For obvious reasons I shall refer mostly to changes in Britain, but I shall draw also on recent developments and experience in the U.S. I suspect that much of what I have to say will be applicable to other countries with differing systems or philosophies of health-care.

There are three major and growing areas through which constraints are being applied to the freedom of doctors - ethical considerations, applications of the law, and the consequences of limited available resources and cost-containment. A fourth category- governmental or authoritarian control - is emerging in Britain through the contents of a White Paper outlining new proposals for managing our Health Service. In many respects these factors have overlapping influences on clinical practice.

Ethics, Law and Medicine

When I first qualified I inherited responsibility for the hospital iron-lung. It was used exclusively for patients with respiratory problems associated with potentially-reversible neurological disease- poliomyelitis or infective polyneuritis. There was no problem about the decision to terminate treatment. The patients were almost always young, their diseases potentially reversible, one made every possible effort to keep them alive. Treatment was stopped when death took place; this moment was recognised by cessation of the heart-beat.

As instrumentation improved the provision of intensive care and life-support systems became cheaper and more readily available. Some of the patients treated in this way had reversible pathology; some had not. A new ethical problem had been created. Even when the outcome was judged to be hopeless, could one switch off a ventilator or cardiac stimulator, withdraw life-support and allow a patient to die? Some patients with profound brain damage, e.g. after cardiac arrest, could be kept in profound coma, in an irreversible vegetative state for many months or years. Such circumstances caused deep distress to their families, were costly, and occupied resources that might have been needed to save the lives of other patients. A new set of criteria, both medical and ethical, were needed to allow the withdrawal of treatment in certain conditions. This led to the development of the concept of brain-death, recognised by death of the brain-stem, which could be established by tests of neurological and respiratory function and which indicated a permanent loss of the capacity for consciousness and for spontaneous respiration. These criteria are now accepted almost universally by doctors in the UK and the considerable experience that has accrued since they were first introduced appears to have vindicated their use.

The medical prerogative to make such decisions has been challenged in many parts of the world. Relatives have begun to exercise what they see as a moral duty to intervene in the interests of the incompetent or unresponsive patient, and many people have expressed their preference for or against such treatment, in advance of an event that might limit their competence to decide. Such advance directives are often formulated in the US through "living wills" which carry moral, if not legal, authority and are usually regarded as helpful to doctors faced with difficult life-or-death decisions. Indeed in some American states such directions are legally enforceable. The choice made by the patient is regarded as the preeminent factor, the role of the physician being to provide appropriate information, perhaps to impart his own judgement or preferences to the patient, but not to make the final decision. In the Netherlands the process has been taken a step further by the introduction of voluntary euthanasia through which a doctor may connive with a patient to end his life when its quality has become intolerable. As we know, this practice is not legally-approved in the Netherlands but is condoned by the lack of litigation against doctors who adopt it.

Such issues raise the wider question of the autonomy of the individual or responsible relatives or guardians to make decisions about medical management. Medical decisions were once quite easily determined; they were made by a doctor and usually accepted without reservation by patients and their families. Today, it is an acknowledged and proper part of good clinical practice to provide as much information to those concerned as might be needed for their informed participation in decision-making. The extent of such information and of their participation is almost certainly greater in the US where patient-rights are a more powerful issue. In the UK difficult ethical decisions about life and death are still traditionally made by doctors, usually after discussion with others familiar with the case-medical and nursing staff and social workers. Doctors generally discuss the decision with relatives but they do not customarily seek the prior opinion or agreement of the patient. In assuming this responsibility doctors have, in general, been guided by humanitarian principles, recognising the extreme difficulty patients and their relatives might experience in such distressing circumstances.

Dunstan uses the term "autonomy", as applied to patients, to embrace two notions: the first is negative, the expression by the patient of a wish not to be treated or operated on without consent; the second is positive, freedom to choose the form and content of treatment without regard to medical or other considerations. The first notion is relatively easy to deal with: whatever moral misgivings a doctor may have about withholding potentially beneficial treatment from a patient who has expressed a desire not to have it, the legal position seems clear - any attempt to impose treatment on a competent patient against his will would constitute an assault. No-one competent can be forced to accept treatment even when doctors are convinced it could be life-saving. What of Dunstan's second notion of autonomy? Do patients ever have positive rights to medical care, to demand specific treatment of their own choosing, or more general intervention such as resuscitation in the event of cardiac arrest? The issue is highlighted by the current debate on abortion in the US. The legal position, in the UK at least, is clear: Doctors are under no legal obligation to offer treatment or carry out investigations they consider unnecessary or harmful. It has, in fact, been established that through our nationalised health service the Government is not legally obliged to provide treatment, even if lifesaving, e.g. renal dialysis for end-stage renal failure.

In all such decisions about life and death and medical intervention there is a delicate interplay between the wishes of patients and their relatives, the law, the ethical values of a particular society, and a doctor's judgement of the correctness of a particular course. This judgement itself, in good medical practice, takes account of humanitarian factors such as the quality of life currently enjoyed and to be anticipated, the social, domestic and psychological background to the illness, and the financial costs to the individual and to Society, usually to the State. In the U.K. this balance is usually tipped in favour of the medical opinion, with an outcome that, I would immodestly suggest, is fair and proper in the vast majority of cases. In the US far greater influence is exerted by patients and their relatives, by the law and, because of the nature of their health-care system, by financial considerations. The status of those who provide care for incompetent patients is far more insecure. This was exemplified in the case of Karen Quinlan, a young girl in a vegetative state, who was being kept alive by artificial mechanical means at great expense and with no hope of recovery. Her parents, devout Catholics, after profound consideration, asked the doctors to remove the ventilator. This they refused to do, partly for moral reasons, partly for concern that they might legally be found guilty of ending Karen's life. Eventually, the New Jersey Supreme Court acknowledged that the girl's father, her doctors and the ethics committee of the hospital could jointly decide whether to withdraw treatment or not.

This eminently sensible decision was rejected by the Massachusetts Court in the Saikewicz case, in which it was asserted that all decisions about the application of life-prolonging measures to terminally-ill incompetent patients was a matter for judicial resolution - "such questions of life and death seem to us to require the detached but passionate investigation and decision of the judicial branch of government". In these terms, doctors were not allowed to exercise their professional judgement. Even urgent decisions had to be deferred for Court approval.

In the UK doctors have been privileged, since the law still recognises and respects the medical role in decisions of a moral or ethical nature, and allows considerable latitude to our professional judgement. In the US this function has to a large extent been taken over by ethicist-philosophers and lawyers. Not only do they enunciate general ethical principles but they now intrude into specific clinical decisions about individual patients.

The prominence of lawyers in such debates and the influence of the legally-respected views of professional ethicists indicates the extent to which moral and ethical issues are decided in the US in the shadow of medical litigation. Its consequences have been profound, affecting almost all doctors. Economically, they are obliged to pay exorbitant premiums (recovered by those in private practice by simply incorporating them into increased charges to their patients); emotionally they suffer the ignominy and trauma of malpractice suits; professionally many have found it advisable to abandon certain procedures, such as obstetrics, or to modify their styles of practice. The adversarial approach has led to an erosion of the relationship between doctors and patients - "Every patient that walks in the door is a potential enemy and a potential litigant".

A most important and serious outcome of litigation is the adoption by most doctors - and indeed most hospitals - of "defensive medicine", through which doctors carry out - or do not carry out - certain procedures, not on the basis of clinical need, but as a defence against potential malpractice charges. The American Medical Association recently estimated that defensive medicine costs annually 15-40 billion dollars, adding about 5% to the total US health-care expenditure.

In the UK we have been spared this awful outcome. A major factor in our health-care system is the buffer provided by the general practitioner who is known personally to his patients, who usually feel well-disposed towards him, and reluctant therefore to litigate. In the more impersonal hospital sector, complaints and litigation are becoming more prevalent, but the absence of a contingency fee payment system removes the positive encouragement to litigate and different methods of assessing damages result in lower awards and, thus, a lessened incentive to sue.

The spectre of litigation constitutes a serious threat to clinical freedom. It encourages patterns of behaviour and decision-taking that are often contrary to best professional judgement; it induces a confrontational attitude of patients towards their doctors which cannot in the longterm be to their benefit. I believe that much of this undesirable litigious activity arises from our own failure to monitor and take steps to improve the quality of care provided by our profession, a theme I shall return to later.

In considering some aspects of clinical practice I

have tried to indicate the conjoint and interrelated influences of ethics and the law, and the ways in which they have begun to impinge on clinical freedom. However unhappy doctors may feel about these emerging constraints, they now readily accept the limitations that are applied to the conduct of medical research. It was not always so. In the first half of the last century doctors assumed a licence to experiment on people and it was not uncommon for institutional inmates to be used for such purposes without any thought of the consequences. William Wallace, a Dublin physician, felt no qualms then about inoculating syphilitic material into five healthy young adults, 19 to 35 years old, long before there was any recognised treatment. By contrast, Neisser, who discovered the gonococcus in 1879, knew that to prove it caused gonorrhoea he would have to demonstrate its infectivity. No animal vectors were known, so the experiment would have to be done in humans. To his great credit, Neisser declined to do this and preferred to remain in doubt. He didn't have to wait long, for within a few years colleagues in Germany had carried out the crucial experiments by successfully inoculating humans with gonorrhoea, thus proving it was transmitted by Neisser's organism.

This cavalier disregard for human rights offended the German public and the government. In 1900 the Prussian Government issued an edict stating that "medical interventions for purposes other than diagnosis, therapy or immunisation are absolutely prohibited ... if the person is a minor or not fully competent ... has not declared his consent unequivocally ... and unless he has had a proper explanation of the adverse consequences that might result" - an admirable sentiment that would stand in any modern-day statement of ethics.

For the subjects of research to be provided with full and proper protection, apart from Governmental edict, a professional conscience had to emerge. This began to appear early in the century and was catapulted into action by the atrocities of Nazi experimentation. Codes of ethical practice of research have now been developed and promulgated in most western countries. On the whole the subjects of research are well-protected and doctors accept constraints on their freedom to experiment with little or no debate. There remain many unresolved issues in the field of research using human subjects but these are complex and varied and will not be further developed here.

Economic constraints

Doctors generate the bulk of medical costs and in most countries are now being asked to be less profligate and to be more accountable. To what extent is this beginning to curtail clinical freedom?

It is not easy to identify or isolate the part played by awareness of cost when individual doctors decide whether or not to investigate or treat individual patients. Faced with, say, an elderly patient who might or might not benefit from chemotherapy or surgery, most doctors would ask themselves, "Is it worth it?" They would be thinking of the pain, discomfort, inconvenience and risk to the patient, rather than money. For practical purposes they would, in the UK at least, be free to prescribe treatment regardless of financial considerations. Those who were persuaded against a particular treatment on financial grounds would not see it as a concession of their clinical freedom, so long as it was their choice. If, however, they were officially prevented from prescribing treatment on the same grounds, they would construe it as a serious curtailment; the decision would have been taken out of their hands.

This is one of the aspects that is of most concern to doctors about the Government's new proposals for the Health Service - the prospect that clinical decisions would be dictated by considerations of cost instead of what was best for the patient. Much of our White Paper reflects the influence of US philosophy about health-care. In it we detect a move towards diagnosis-related groups (DRGs) through which payments will be made to hospitals according to the category of the patient's illness. General practitioners will be given fixed budgets with which to purchase hospital or community care for their patients and "will need to be aware in advance of the consequences for the budget of referral to hospital". Hospitals will have to fix the prices of the facilities they offer and compete against one another for GP referrals; "the hospital bears the cost (or reaps the benefit) if outcome costs differ from assessed costs".

In this scheme of things the cost of investigations and treatment will have a dominant influence on clinical decisions, and it is not difficult to foresee a situation in which a doctor will be obliged to refuse or limit treatment to a particular patient because his budget does not permit it. When DRGs were introduced in the US, Eli Ginzberg remarked "the earlier untramelled freedom of the profession to determine how, where and for how long patients would be treated was being circumscribed by new rules, regulations and protocols". What has happened in the US, looks set to happen in Britain.

It is abundantly clear that no system of healthcare can continue to offer the best possible medical services to all of its people all of the time. Some form of rationing is inevitable. Professor Rudolf Klein distinguishes between macro-rationing and micro-rationing, the former dependent on national or regional policy decisions about the allocation of recources, the latter concerned with the fine detail of which patient receives what treatment. This distinction highlights the dilemma faced by doctors who deal directly with patients and who are required to recognise their responsibility to Society as well as to their patients. In doing so, they may accept the generalisation that obtaining scarce resources for one patient reduces their availability to others, but this does not make it any easier when dealing with a particular individual to withhold potentially beneficial treatment on the grounds of cost or scarcity. Some years ago in my own city of Birmingham the local Health Authority imposed a limit on the number of patients to be admitted to a renal dialysis programme. This led to vigorous protest during the course of which the question was asked whether a doctor could ever allow a patient to die of a treatable disorder because he is ordered to do so by the State.

The imposition of rationing, the allocation of financial or other resources between regions of a country or between different disciplines, is an authoritarian decision; implementation of these decisions at the point of contact between doctor and patient is a personal and intimate act which may run contrary to the whole professional ethos. In Britain we are now seeing an attempt by Government to set targets which it expects doctors to achieve. In the US, through Health Maintenance Organisations (HMOs) a similar approach is already manifest. Within HMOs doctors are subject to regular review which embraces the number of patients they see each day, how many are admitted and for how long, their use of investigative facilities, their prescription patterns, the rates at which they refer patients to specialists, even their teaching and research activities. A Republican Senator, J John Heinz III of Pennsylvania, remarked that hospitals were "pressing doctors to violate their own medical judgement in treating patients", and that some "publicly rank the performance of their doctors, with good marks and even financial bonuses going to those with shorter stay, money-saving patients, and black marks for those with the sicker, older "DRG losers."

The US approach and the threatened UK approach incorporate elements that seriously erode clinical freedom. Are they wholly unreasonable? Can any Government or employing institution accept an open-ended arrangement through which doctors are permitted to consume resources without constraints? Should any doctor be free to prescribe expensive antibiotics at public expense when cheaper ones would do? Or expensive chemotherapy for tumours that are unlikely to respond? To offer surgery when the benefits of that operation have not clearly been demonstrated? Clinical freedom that permits the thoughtless and wasteful use of recources cannot be defended. I believe it is the responsibility of the medical profession to ensure that such extravagance is curtailed. Good sense and wisdom in the use of recources is an integral part of good clinical practice and, as a profession, we should insist upon it.

Improving standards by medical audit

I have described various trends towards a diminution of the clinical freedom of doctors-ethical and legal considerations, public pressures and, above all, financial constraints. If we wish to preserve those elements of clinical freedom that we regard as important, we must do all in our power to improve the standards of medical care and of professional performance. The term Medical Audit (or its various euphemisms) is used to include a number of related but different activities. At one end of the range are those processes that examine how our facilities are being used - bed occupancy rates, outpatient waiting lists, the use of operating theatres, X-ray or other diagnostic equipment. Such activities are needed to optimise the use of resources; they are predominantly managerial but depend on appropriate medical advice and collaboration. Two elements of audit are essentially our concern as doctors:

First is a proper study of the outcome of our interventions. Medicine is full of unresolved controversies: Who should have regular serum cholesterol tests? Or cervical screening? Or mammography? Is there a place for regular screening of healthy individuals? Should all patients with stroke have a CT scan? Or all patients with head injuries a skull X-ray? One can go on and on. Until we resolve such controversies we cannot discuss optimal management - and we cannot be serving the interests of our patients - or our Governments- properly. I hope the profession will increasingly devote itself to outcome studies that may provide sound guidance to our future practitioners.

Second is our need to monitor and, hence, improve the quality of care provided by our profession. Serious deficiencies and serious misconduct are usually dealt with by a variety of statutory bodies, in Britain by the General Medical Council. We too readily tolerate lesser degress of competence amongst our colleagues. Without making any objective analysis, most doctors have a pretty good idea about the quality of care offered by other doctors. We recognise good medical practitioners - and bad ones. General practitioners tend to refer their patients to specialists they recognise as providers of high quality care. We all know which of our colleagues to call in when we need help, especially when we or our families need attention.

This sort of appraisal can - and should - be formalised. The Royal College of Physicians of London has recently published a report on Medical Audit which advises all hospitals to establish systems for assessing the individual medical management of individual patients. The case-notes of recently- discharged patients will be scrutinised to assess the standard of note-keeping, to ensure that all information is clearly recorded including what the patients and relatives have been told about the illness, and to ensure that the discharge-letter and case-summary have been expeditiously completed and dispatched. Apart from this, consultants and their junior staff are expected to attend regular meetings (once a week, preferably) at which selected case- notes will be reviewed and details of management critically discussed. This type of meeting conforms to a system set up more than ten years ago by the Academic (Professorial) Medical Department in Birmingham, of which I was Chairman, which had a noticeable beneficial effect on standards of practice and on the way in which doctors think about their actions. We found that the most important questions to ask were of the form of "Why was such-and-such a test performed?" or "Why was that treatment chosen instead of another?" Such questions forced the subject of review to justify his actions, to explain why he had chosen a particular course of action, and very rapidly led to a change of attitude on the wards, where a marked decline was noted in the number of investigations ordered (especially as an emergency) and in the number of medicines prescribed - without, we have good reason to believe, any deterioration in the quality of care given to our patients.

In the US, Peer Review organisations have extended their interest from cost-control to clinical competence, examining such aspects as unexplained hospital readmissions soon after discharge, medical or surgical mishaps, adverse drug reactions, faulty diagnoses and unnecessary admissions. The performance of individual doctors as well as individual institutions is increasingly subject to surveillance.

In Britain a recent report of the Royal College of Surgeons, the Confidential Enquiry into Postoperative Deaths, found great variation between mortality rates for standard operations between different hospitals in different parts of the country. What was most disturbing was their revelation that about 20% of all deaths were due to avoidable surgical or anaesthetic causes. This is not a circumstance that we, as doctors, should tolerate.

Our profession has the authority to exert a profound influence on the lives of individuals; in some situations, to confer life or deliberately to end it. By our carelessness or negligence or mismanagement we may cause it to end prematurely. Some scrutiny of our competence to bear such great responsibility should not be construed as an enchroachment on our authority. We should welcome it, indeed insist on it, for only by such scrutiny can we lay any claim to the preservation of the clinical freedom we so fortunately still enjoy.

Acknowledgement

This paper is based on a monograph prepared during tenure of a Rock-Carling Fellowship of the Nuffield Provincial Hospitals Trust and published by them in 1987.

CLINICAL FREEDOM: PATIENTS' AND PHYSICIANS' AUTONOMY VERSUS THE DEMANDS OF SOCIETY

Povl Riis

Clinical freedom as a term seems to be self-explanatory to many doctors, and even heavily loaded with positive values. Still, a thorough analysis of the term needs to start with defining the two words, **clinical** and **freedom**.

Clinical is the easiest to define in accordance with present-time semantics: all procedures and circumstances related to the patient-doctor-relationship, whether in general practice, in a hospital set-up, or in acute, non-institutionalized situations.

Freedom elicits less consensus in semantics. Here it is defined as the sum of personal choices, experienced by an individual.

Autonomy as an ethical key-word

Autonomy, i.e. the right to self-determination, is a fundamental concept within the universe of basic human rights. Without autonomy most of such rights have no meaning. The right to express one's views in speech or print does not exist, if the views expressed are not founded on an autonomous choice. The same is true for the freedom of faith.

Autonomy is however only a **necessary**, and not a **sufficient** condition for creating and stimulating a collectivity, whether in a national or a global perspective. In other words, a democratic society with welfare responsibilities towards its citizens can not be founded on autonomy alone, even if the individual citizen's autonomy serves a voluntary reduction of self-centered interests. Stages of human life, as early childhood and late-in-life dementia, besides transient phases of incompetence due to intoxications, head traumata etc., create a need for motive forces, supplementary to autonomy. The supplement can be a delegated autonomy to relatives, whether expressed in a living will, or implicitly functioning through family relations. Or leaving the person-to-person level, states can reduce autonomy of citizens as in obligatory military services (only to be suspended in open democratic societies in cases of conscientious objection), and states and governments can exclude tax-paying from the spheres of personal autonomy - and do it!

The complimentarity of freedom and autonomy

In a societal context no one can possess freedom, defined as the sum of choices, without reducing other persons' sum of choices, at least when the freedom of the first person reaches a certain level. Thus, freedom and restrictions are complementary in a person-to-person and a person-to-society universe. The same is true for autonomy in similar universes, the right to self-determination being complementary to the loss of self-determination of others, because multiple expressions of autonomy in a closed universe are mutually competitive, at least beyond a minimal level.

The same complementarity holds true for duties and rights. No one can possess rights without others having duties, and vice versa. Again, this is obvious in inter-personal relations, but even in person-to-society relations, when the universe is the open democratic society. Here a basic philosophy of justice and fairness makes it similarly impossible to imagine that individual citizens or groups of citizens can claim to possess rights without duties, even if such a complementarity is not based on inborn laws of logic, but is politically determined.

Economy and resource aspects

Turning to economics and non-economic resources, as organs for transplantation and very specialized professional manpower, one again meets the complementarity. Every decision of spending money or resources means the exclusion of other spending purposes.

Within the health professions this basic complementarity of spending, and excluding alternative choices, has arrived very late. In a context of clinical freedom it means, that money and non-financial resources link clinical decisions to a number of non-decisions in the closed universe of a societal health system.

Legal regulations

Even if most legal regulations are restrictive of nature, they are still parts of a complementary system, represented by citizens' expectations, or even what citizens consider to be obvious human rights. This is especially true in non-democratic societies. But also open democratic societies know of such complementary relations. If a society does not accept brain-death as a legal death criterion, the citizen with a severe cardiomyopathy, being prevented from getting access to heart transplantation, will feel that the law reduces his or her right to life-saving medical help. Similarly the woman facing a non-wanted pregnancy, will feel that her autonomy and freedom is severly restricted in countries without a Free Abortion Act. Sanctions linked to such restrictive laws will further increase the citizens' feelings of a reduced sum of personal choices.

Applying concepts and analyses to clinical situations

The key-terms and analytic techniques will consequently have to be applied to important fields within the spectrum of clinical situations. The fields are the following:
- daily clinical work, with an obvious possibility of benefiting the patient
- marginal clinical situations, with a very doubtful (or "non-existing") benefit for the patient
- research, involving patients
- health education, involving patients.

1. Daily clinical work

The majority of clinical situations in peacetime, includes an obvious possibility of benefiting the patient, applying interventions, that are accepted by the autonomous patient (and relatives), by the clinician, and which belong to the feasible armamentarium of he country in question (Fig.1). In such situations clinical freedom is in fact existing, seen from both the patient's and the clinician's point-of-view. If however the patient turns down all therapeutic suggestions (even if they could be life-saving), or if he or she suggests an intervention that is unacceptable to the clinician, the patient's refusal will have to be respected, and the same is true on the doctor's side, with an additional obligation for her or him to arrange a second opinion contact with another institution or clinician.

Figure 1   Flow chart - daily clinical work

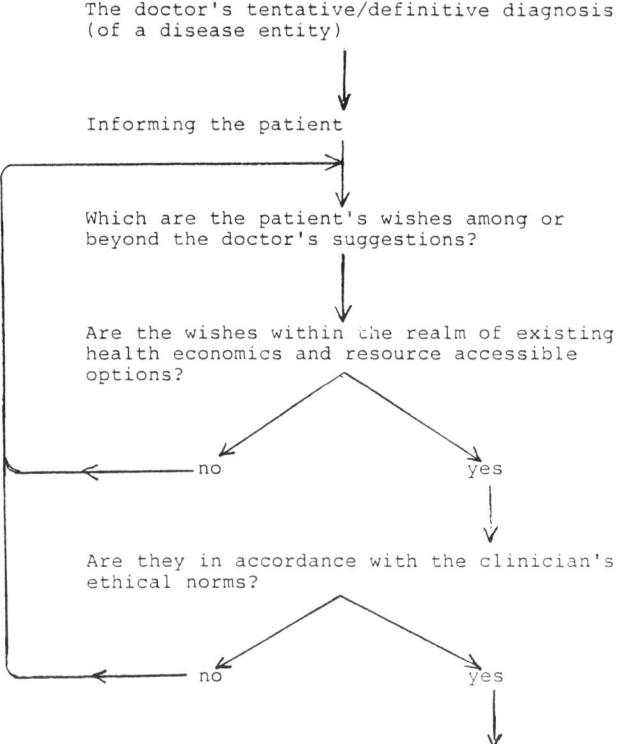

If both the patient and the doctor agrees on the therapeutic choice, but if this choice is <u>not</u> accessible in the country, neither for the given patient, nor for anyone else (for instance chronic haemodialysis, heart transplantation etc.), the clinical freedom is reduced, and the hard facts of health economy and politics step in.

2. Marginal clinical situations

All clinical decision making now and then comprises situations, where the clinical freedom is reduced, due to the existence of only few and doubtful therapeutical options in a given situation, for instance dealing with the very old and/or desperately ill patient (Fig.2). Here the clinician's knowledge of prognostic indicators from clinical research is crucial. Further, dilemmas can arise, if the patient's autonomy is unexpressed, is expressed only through reports of the relatives, or through a - sometimes rather outdated - living will, and if discrepancies between these sources of information and decision making arise. Even the situation, that the clinician exerts his or her right to autonomy in refusing to accept an intervention against personal norms, will appear now and then. Here the clinician has the duty to listen, to scrutinize, and to inform, but at the same time has the right to refuse delivering treatment (again after having arranged for referral to a different institution etc., if at all possible). In such cases, where both parts' autonomy and complementary rights and duties are at a collision course, it will often be helpful to involve an independent institution, as an institutional ethical review board and/or a state medical officer or a judge.

3. Research involving patients

Clinical freedom in a hypothetical world without clinical and fundamental research would be permanently restricted. This situation is clearly illustrated in nations and larger regions of the world, where

Figure 2

<u>Flow chart - marginal clinical situations</u>

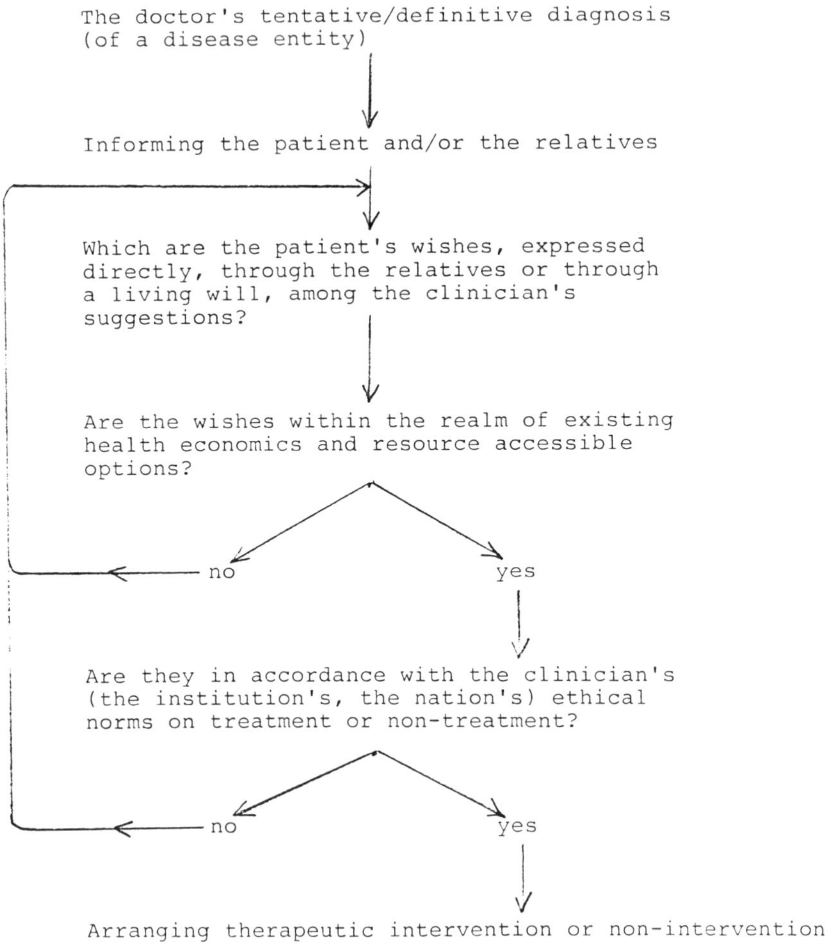

The doctor's tentative/definitive diagnosis
(of a disease entity)
↓
Informing the patient and/or the relatives
↓
Which are the patient's wishes, expressed
directly, through the relatives or through
a living will, among the clinician's
suggestions?
↓
Are the wishes within the realm of existing
health economics and resource accessible
options?

← no   yes →
         ↓
Are they in accordance with the clinician's
(the institution's, the nation's) ethical
norms on treatment or non-treatment?

← no   yes →
         ↓
Arranging therapeutic intervention or non-intervention

biomedical research does not exist, whether for economic or political reasons. Without biomedical research no progress (which is often forgotten by people critisizing modern research, even if they strongly benefit from many decennia's research in their daily life).

The patient and the healthy volunteer have an obvious right to autonomy, by demanding the necessary information and consequently saying yes or no to participation. But all patients do not have the right to use their autonomy to say no to all biomedical projects, if they at the same time demand progress of clinicians and other health workers.

On the other hand the scientist, if all ethical guidelines and national laws are followed strictly, has a right to autonomously expressing his intellectual and health-professional incentive to plan and carry through research projects.

The guidelines and the operational flow-chart applied are well adjusted to biomedical research today (Fig. 3).

Respect for the interaction between citizens' and researchers' rights and duties can be underlined by for instance an obligatory feed-back information to patients after the trial has been completed, informing them on active or placebo treatment, overall results, and consequences for their future treatment. In other words, the delicate multiple interactions between duties and rights known from common human relationships (as friendships, marriages, occupational teamwork etc.) can be applied to research situations, involving human subjects, with great benefit.

4. Education involving patients

As is true for research and progress, education in medicine without access to patients would imply stagnation. As in research situations one can still meet public opinion makers that seem to consider research and teaching in medicine to take place anywhere else, i.e. in places where they do not risk to be involved. Such over-emphasis on autonomy leads to ethnic or geographical egoism, even with the time dimension: historical egoism (forgetting how many of to-day's possibilities in therapeutics were actually created by previous generations' altruistic participation in controlled clinical trials etc.).

Figure 3   Flow chart - research situations

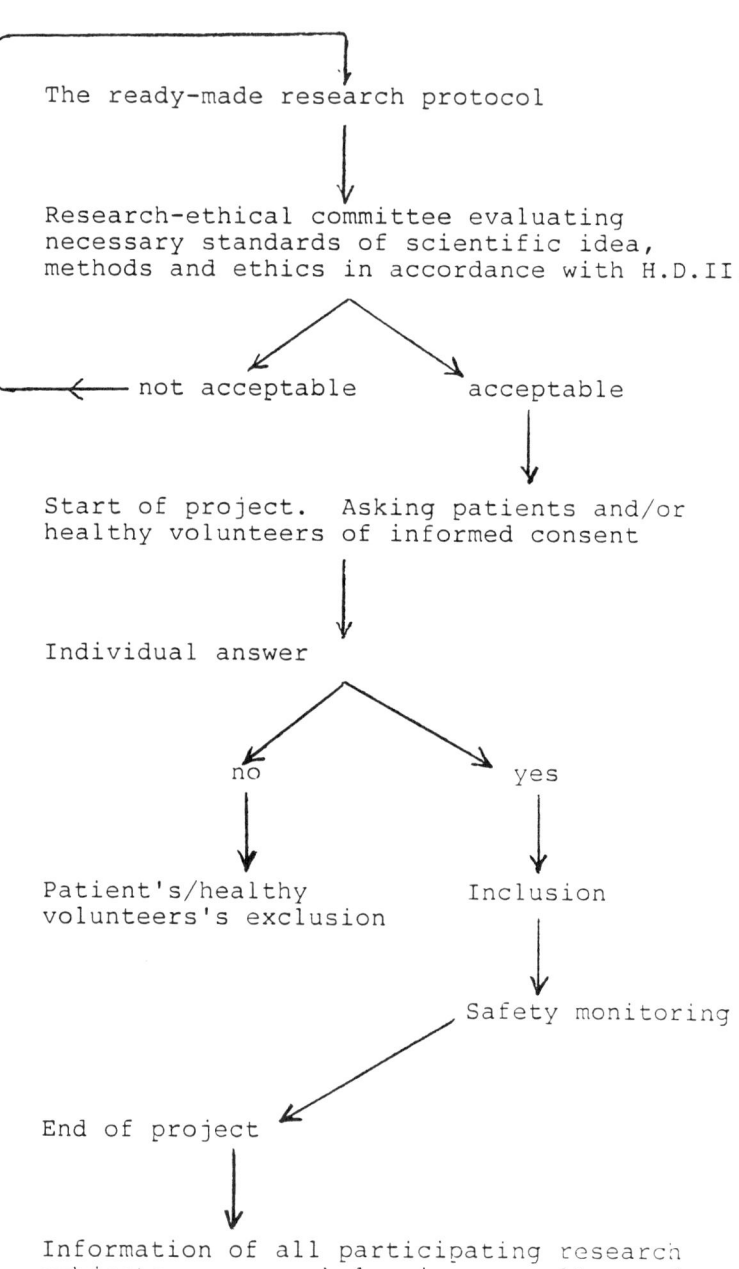

Figure 4   Flow chart - education involving patients

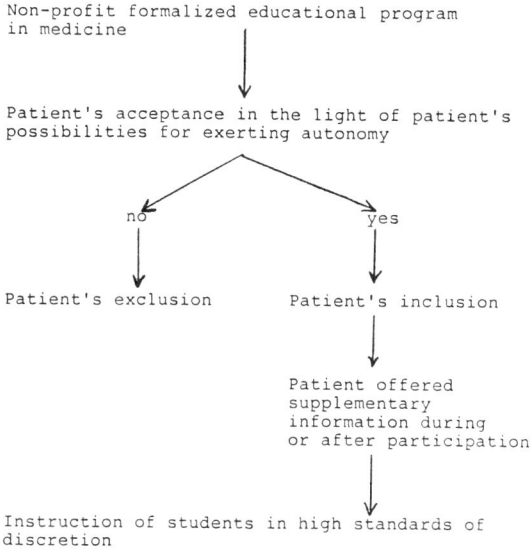

As is shown in Fig.4 patients' participation presupposes certain rules of the game including not only patients' autonomy, but also their integrity, that is the complex of personal norms and the overall self-esteem.

In certain cases, psychotic states, severe intoxications etc., clinical teaching and demonstration is ethically complex. Primary concern will have to be taken to the patient, who might not be able to consent in a meaningful way. Clandestine demonstration via one-way glass walls is no acceptable solution. Sometimes the freedom to select the best possible educational material collides strongly with the patient's interests, always to be given the highest priority. In such cases the solution might be to let actors play the schizophrenic, the paranoic, the manic (etc.) behaviour on video.

Conclusion

The concept "clinical freedom" involves not only the patient and the doctor (as some clinicians still think), but also the institutions, the law, the political decision makers and the assisting health economists. Among these the politicians, besides being responsible for laws and economics, will have to reflect ethical norms prevalent in the population.

The key-words of contemporary ethical discussions, autonomy and paternalism, are insufficient as the conceptual framework for ethical analyses of clinical freedom and scientific freedom. The same is true for "one-sided" application of rights and duties.

All these terms are complementary. Autonomy and respect for autonomy do not meet the demands of a collectivity, forming the base of a modern democratic welfare society. Paternalism is neither a purely negative concept. No citizen can decide only for autonomy, because the selfishness built-in prevents the "loving paternalism" filling any non-autonomous vacuum, where people seem to be in trouble, needing spontaneous man-to-man interventions, not to be postponed during discussions on autonomy.

The extension of autonomy to relatives, or in a written form through living wills, represents a safeguard for patients and research subjects. However, rigid emphasis on informed consent in acute or marginal situations as superior to trust (or clinical freedom in the interest of patients) creates a serious obstacle to the humanitarian perspectives of clinical work and promising research.

Serious reductions of clinical freedom do not always lead to a corresponding increase in patients' freedom, but can instead reduce the possibilities for fulfilling patients' expectations of health and progress.

In other words, patients' sum of choices (=freedom) can in principle be increased as a right to choose, but at the same time be reduced <u>de facto,</u> because less options remain for the choices.

For these reasons clinical freedom is so valuable, not primarily for clinicians, but on the contrary for those that they serve.

<u>References</u>

1. Riis, P.: The necessity and the insufficiency of medical scientific progress. In: Lanza R (ed.). Medical science and the advancement of world health. New York: Praeger, 1985.

2. Riis, P.: Medicinsk videnskabsetik. In: Andersen D, Mabeck CE, Riis P (eds.). Medicinsk etik. Copenhagen: FADL, 1987.

3. Riis, P.: Paternalisme og autonomi - er den etiske rangstilling oplagt? Teol Forum 1989; 2: 3-4.

4. Riis, P., & al.: The Appleton Consensus: Suggested International Guidelines for Decisions to Forgo Medical Treatment. Ugeskr Laeger 1989; 151: 700-6.

Ethics in Medicine, edited by
Peter Allebeck and Bengt Jansson.
Raven Press, New York © 1990.

ON DOCTORS AND PATIENTS

Amnon Carmi

The doctor - patient system of relations is formed by various factors: The two parties, external elements: political, social and economic, and the contact per se - its aim and its nature. Each factor is relevant, the accumulative weight of all factors carries particular significance. The following notes will deal only with a few normative aspects.

The main aim of the doctor - patient contact is to cure the patient. Due to the variety of the external factors, one may notice secondary aims too. For example: The state might be interested in the good health of its citizens, due to security or economic reasons; The society might be interested to adopt- or reject - alternative medicine, etc.

Our discussion will consider the duties and the rights of both physicians and patients in the light of the controversial views with regard to paternalism and autonomy. Apparently, one of the most pervasive and perplexing moral dilemmas in health care is brought into being when the moral principles of benefiting the patient and of respecting the patient's autonomy cross each other.

The term "autonomy" - self rule or self determination - is drawn from the political sphere, where it refers to the independence of states, their rule without external interference. The metaphorical use of this term with regard to the doctor - patient relation has brought about misunderstanding and sharp disputes.

The term "paternalism" is drawn from the role of the father in the family. It shows the claim or attempt to supply the needs or to regulate the life of a cummunity in the same way as a father does with regard to his children.

Paternalism is wrong where the doctor treats the patient as a child, i.e. as one who has not yet freely and competently, and with adequate information, formed a conception of good and evil or benefits and harms, or is not able to act on that conception in these circumstances. There is a bit of hypocrisy in the use of the equation of patient autonomy in contrast to doctor's paternalism.

Take for example the distorted conception of informed consent, which seems to be a queer legalistic product. The process of negotiating between the physician and the patient has been placed and presented upside down. Eventually, it is the patient who asks for the physician's help, and the latter who consents to render his services. The doctor - patient interaction constitutes a bilateral process, the wills of both parties must meet and form an agreement. Both parties discuss the details and exchange pieces of relevant information. The medical treatment reflects a later phase of the whole process.

The successful outcome depends on the commitment of each party to supply the other with a certain amount of data, and requires that both sides are competent and act freely.

The one-sided presentation of the issue, emphasizing only the need for the informed consent of the patient, shows the sociopsychological factors in the historical development of the informed consent theory. Bilateral justice should be shown while interpreting bilateral agreement. Life needs and circumstances require that mutual consideration and concession been shown throughout the doctor - patient interaction in order to settle disputes in a satisfactory manner.

The goal of this interaction is to cure the patient, but the benefit should be granted to the doctor as well.

Thus, one should not disregard societal paternalism towards physicians by issue of licences, socialization of the profession or determining legal and ethical norms.

The art of medicine imposes heavy demands on its practitioners. No wonder that physicians suffer greatly the pains of perplexity.

Judges encounter same dilemmas. The Talmud asks: "Lest the judge say: Why should I have all this trouble?" And the Talmud replies: "He is with you in giving judgement... for the judge there is nothing but that which his eyes perceive".

The same applies to doctors who, like judges, deal with matters of death and life. For them too there is nothing but that which their eyes perceive, and He is with them as they perform their sacred mission of saving human life.

The obligation of the doctor to cure the patient might be founded on legal or sociological conceptions, on moral considerations or regligious belief.

The Halacha provides us with various reasons for the duty of the doctor to treat patients: "Neither shall thou stand idly by the blood of thy fellow" shows that saving life constituted an important commandment in the Torah, binding everyone to do his utmost for lifesaving of his neighbor.

If the doctor withholds his services he is regarded as shedding blood. The obligation of the physician to heal is also inherented in another commandment: "Thou shall love thy neighbor as thyself" (Leviticus 19:18).

Some of the leading scholars, notably Maimonides, conclude that healing the sick is not only allowed but is actually obligatory.

Since the Jewish law requires, as will be later shown, that the patient apply to the doctor, and allows the doctor to treat the patient, this permission to treat becomes an obligation to do so.

The doctor is authorized to treat the patient even if the latter refuses to be treated.

The Supreme Court of Israel has recently ruled in a criminal case, that doctors are entitled to treat (adult and sober) patients even against their will in an emergency situation or where danger is imminent to the patient's health.

A somewhat similat attitude, though not for religious reason, has been adopted by Chinese society (R. Veatach, R. Branson, Ethics and Health Policy, 1976, 57).

The Chinese health care system illustrates a blend of responsibility on the part of the individual to protect his own health and that of his neighbors, and of societal responsibility for nationwide well-being. Health care activity represents a complex mix of decisions made by individuals themselves, and decisions made at a series of organized societal levels.

The roles of the patient and the doctor in Chinese society can be understood only within the Chinese context. Individualism never occupied the central position in China that it has in the west for the past several hundred years. From the Chinese point of view, freedom is not the first concern, and individualism is regarded as selfishness.

Both during their training period and afterward, doctors are exhorted to put the needs of the patient and the need of society ahead of their own preferences.

Physicians have been encouraged to develop more egalitarian relationships with other health workers and with patients in order to maximize the effectiveness of every individual. They even try to follow life styles that will not distinguish them from the others. A startling example occured during the Cultural Revolution, when publication of all scientific journals was suspended in order to reduce the use of these journals for the fame and gain of the authors.

Coming back to the Jewish religious tradition, physicians are bound to treat also poor patients who are not able to pay the medical fees, and doctors are expected to render their services even where the treatment is beneath their professional status or dignity.

Let us now turn to the patient and examine his legal, ethical and religious duties.

In Jewish law and moral teaching the value of human life is supreme and takes precedence over virtually all other considerations.

Human life is not a good to be preserved as a condition of other values but an absolute basic and precious good in its own stead. The obligation to preserve life is all-encompassing.

The Law of Moses is the Law of life, hence its concern for health. Every one must refrain from hurting his neighbor or himself, and each should receive medical treatment.

Maimonides claimed that the stupid pious who refuses medical aid and relies only on the heavenly help, reminds him of the hungry man who rejects the bread and prays to God in order to be cured from the disease of hunger.

The following story illustrates the implementation of this conception (Berakhot 5 b):

Rabbi Yohanan once fell ill and Rabbi Hanina went to visit him saying: "Are your sufferings welcome to you?" Rabbi Yohanan replied: "Neither they nor their reward", implying that one who lovingly accepts sufferings in this world will be greatly compensated in the world to come. Rabbi Hanina then said: "Give me your hand", which Rabbi Yohanan did, and he cured him. Why could not Rabbi Yohanan cure himself, asks the Talmud. The reply is "Beacuse the prisoner cannot free himself from jail", meaning the patient cannot cure himself.

The Sages forbade people to live in any city which had no physicians. According to the Halacha, man does not posses absolute title to his life or to his body. Title to human life is vested in the Creator, and man is but the steward of the life which he has been privileged to receive. Therefore, man is charged with preserving, dignifying and hallowing that life. When falling victim to illness he is obliged to seek a cure in order to sustain life.

Coming back to the Chinese socialistic approach, patients are expected to participate in their own care. The patient's initiative is needed to fight the disease. Education and persuation are used in order to advance the public interest and knowledge.

How should we settle the dispute between all these conflicting interests and conceptions?

First of all, society should reconsider and reshape its attitude toward the commonly abused medical profession.

R. Yehuda claimed: Most of donkey drivers are wicked, most of camel drivers are honest, most of sailors are honest, the best of physicians deserves hell (Mishna Kidushin 84:14). Bernard Shaw claimed: Doctors are just like other Englishmen: Most of them have no honour and no conscience (The Doctor's Dilemma, preface on doctors).

How come? The embroidery of medicine has been woven into Jewish thought since ever. The Jewish Sages treated medicine with deep respect and high appreciation, and many of the Jewish leaders wear both crowns of Torah and medicine.

Bernard Shaw claimed: "The butcher and the baker are not expected to feed the hungry unless the hungry can pay; but a doctor who allows a fellow - creature to suffer or perish without aid is regarded as a monster". He added: "The doctor is, by the nature of his work, an emergency man. A doctor is expected to work day and night, and to the strain of such inhuman conditions must be added the constant risk of infection".

In short, the doctor needs our help much more than we often need his.

The present dispute involves strong arguments and obvious emotional reactions with regard to dignity and freedom and the right of self determination. According to the Jewish tradition, God created man and woman in His own image, which in itself makes for human dignity as the reflected splendour of divine dignity. Dignity means merit or worth. It includes recognition of one's worth both by others and by one's self. Respect means recognizing the worth and the rights of others, and regarding each individual as equal to every other. Dignity serves as a substantial component of human behavior in society.

In our case it will be respected only if both the physician and the patient will commmit themselves.

A social recognition of an individual's entitlement to make certain choices is a symbolic expression of respect for persons. There is a value attached to a person's freedom to make important choices, and to a person's entitlement to make such choices.

According to Judaism men are considered as a unique species because they enjoy the free choice and they are the only ones who are capable to distinguish between good and evil. Being human necessarily means to become free. The important factor is, that as a free person man is expected to bear the burden of responsibility.

According to an old legend, when pregnancy occurs, the Angel lifts up a drop, places it in front of God and makes his enquiry: "Master of the world, what should become out of the drop - a hero or a weak person? A wise man or a fool? A rich man or a poor one?"

However, the Master will never determine whether the new born will be righteous or wicked, as the newborn will be entitled to make his own choice in his right time: "All is foreseen, but the freedom of choice is given".

Freedom does not mean anarchy. To become free means to bear responsibility, the responsibility for making choice, the choice which takes into consideration _all_ interests involved.

What we need and look for is that kind of negotiation which will help us to build a normative system, the nature of which will not be paternalistic or autonomous per se, but a satisfactory product of the joint effort to bear responsibility throughout the healing process.

Ethics in Medicine, edited by
Peter Allebeck and Bengt Jansson.
Raven Press, New York © 1990.

ETHICAL PROBLEMS IN EPIDEMIOLOGICAL RESEARCH

INTRODUCTION

Claes-Göran Westrin

The title of the subject at issue in this section may sound somewhat sophisticated but it is in fact an issue in focus of the public interest. An example of this is a placard recently from a respected newspaper, the conservative Svenska Dagbladet:

> RESEARCHERS PROVOKE
> THOUSANDS OF TWINS
> WITH INTIMATE QUESTIONS

The story referred to concerned an epidemiological study of mental health problems in a Swedish population.

Attention like this is not unusual for Swedish epidemiologists. This may from one aspect be welcome - it shows that epidemiology is an active and important area in the community. Nevertheless, it is not something which make us very happy and there is a very evident explanation why. In all these stories we are almost always given the role of the villain; the dangerous Big Brother who sees and controls everything, a Peeping Tom or at best an irritating bore. This image of epidemiological research seems also to have markedly reduced the traditionally very good conditions for epidemiological research in Sweden- with increasing attrition rates, legal and other difficulties in record linkage etc.

We have also - of course - some difficulties to accept the roles we have been bestowed. We can for example hardly see ourselves as more villainous than the journalists, who also have their computerized case registers, not only to use in anonymous analyses of groups but actually for control of and information about identified individuals.

We can also refer to a satisfactory record concerning the standard of confidentiality during decades and decades of epidemiological research.

Thus, ethical risks in case register research do not seem to deserve the attacks, not even the interest, which have made them a central ethical issue in the Swedish debate.

However, epidemiologists are increasingly aware of many other ethical problems in epidemiological research and practice. Attempts have also been made in the International Epidemiological Association (IEA) as well as in this country to set up ethical guidelines for epidemiologists. We are very happy to have a contribution from John M Last who is coordinator of the IEA work - as we are happy to have been able to recruit a very competent panel to comment on his current concepts and other questions of this important aspect of public health research.

AN ETHICAL FRAMEWORK FOR EPIDEMIOLOGY

John M. Last

Epidemiology presents issues in ethics and social policy that resemble those of public health: the needs of society can have higher priority than the rights of individuals. This accords with the utilitarian philosophial concept of achieving the greatest good for the greatest number. Judged by the published record, biomedical ethics has not been much concerned with issues arising in public health or epidemiology, but several problems have become prominent in recent years.

Whether conducting surveillance or research, epidemiologists deal with the general public, i.e., free-living people in the community; and with sick people or patients. Either members of the public or patients may be research subjects. Epidemiologists also deal with health administrators and policy makers, research granting agencies, the media, special interest groups of many kinds; and usually with an employer. Interacting with all these groups, epidemiologists adhere to the same principles and moral values as biomedical practitioners and scientists in other fields.

Epidemiologists and epidemic disease

Two ancient customs that gave rise to rules about contagion were present at the creation of epidemiology. In biblical times, lepers carried a bell to warn others of their coming; and since the 14th century, ships and those who sailed in them have been subject to quarantine. Laws evolved from these customs and the laws have consequences: they can lead to stigmatizing and ostracizing of persons with contagious disease, and to restriction of freedom.

These consequences were tolerated until the AIDS epidemic led to over-reactions, widely publicized abuses, and well-organized resistance by stigmatized groups. The issues here have less to do with ethics than with emotional influences on social policy; they have been exhaustively discussed in many countries, but no clear consensus has emerged: instead, locally prevailing values have often been invoked to set policies that can vary even within different sections of the same administrative and political jurisdiction. Similar but less extreme variations in policy influence other aspects of epidemiological practice and research.

Ethics and the science of epidemiology

When conducting research, epidemiologists can encounter moral and ethical minefields: in dealing with human subjects, in defining obligations and responsibilities to various interest groups, in relation to the ownership of the data generated in studies, and in the presentation of research results. It has been suggested that guidelines or a code of conduct may help us deal with some of the moral ambiguities.

Several professional organizations of epidemiologists have considered what should be included in guidelines or a code. As a Council member of the International Epidemiological Association, I have been responsible for drafting and circulating a statement about guidelines on ethics for epidemiologists, and for attempting to collate responses into a coherent document.

The first draft of this document was circulated in January 1988; it was continuing to elicit reactions twenty months later, suggesting that it provoked a good deal of thought. This document defines epidemiology and specifies its purposes; it outlines the basic principles of biomedical ethics; it includes clauses dealing with the ethics of informed consent, privacy and confidentiality, impartiality and objectivity (and their antonym, conflict of interest), with truth-telling and scientific honesty, and with cultural differences and their implications. In short, it spells out duties to all of the groups and individuals with whom epidemiologists work.

Responsibilities to research subjects

Epidemiologists, like other biomedical scientists, honour the Helsinki Declaration, which upholds the principle of autonomy or respect for human dignity and freedom, and outlines acceptable standards for medical research involving human objects. One important safeguard for research subjects is the requirement to obtain their informed consent before conducting research on them. This requirement is explicitly stated in many national guidelines or codes of ethics dealing with medical research. But informed consent is neither simple nor straightforward, as numerous discussions and publications make abundantly clear.

Ethics review committees and research granting agencies usually insist on compliance with formal procedures for obtaining informed consent. This sometimes creates onerous duties for clinical research workers. The progress of randomized controlled trials may be impeded if ethics review committees insist upon communication of such minatory detail that potential research subjects are frightened off. For example, investigators planning a randomized controlled trial of breast cancer treatment methods, reacting to their perception of the granting agency's rules, composed a consent form reading roughly as follows: "I understand that I have breast cancer; I understand that there is uncertainty about the best way to treat my disease; with this understanding, I consent to allow the method of treatment in my case to be determined by chance." Consultations between the investigators and the ethics review committee contributed to the composition of a more softly worded consent form.

There are uncertainties about proxy consent: this can come from parents or responsible close kin of mentally incompetent adults - or from a physician-superintendent in loco parentis. There are uncertainties about so-called "partial" consent. The process itself raises questions - by whom is consent obtained, is it truly informed, is it truly voluntary, are there threats, bribery? Were potential research subjects manipulated? There are important cultural variations in perception of autonomy: some patients regard their doctor as the decision-maker, in some societies, a religious or tribal leader makes decisions for followers.

The rigorous requirements of ethics review committees can cause difficulties for epidemiologists, for example if the research involves gathering information from large existing data files. Policies and practice on access vary among the nations that have such data files. To what extent does a consent form permit the study of personal details not mentioned at the time persons sign this form? They may have signed a vaguely worded consent form months or years earlier than the time that research workers want to study their records, e.g., when they entered hospital, enrolled in a health insurance program, or obtained employment in an industry with its own health service. Here the question of informed consent merges with the issues that arise in protecting privacy and confidentiality.

Privacy and confidentiality

Respect for the privacy and confidentiality of research subjects also follows from the principle of autonomy. Privacy may be invaded, confidentiality violated by inadvertently releasing or publishing information that can identify a person, or even, in some circumstances, a community. When inhabitants of a certain community objected to this being identified as the "unhealthiest" town in the nation (1), some of my colleagues had to conduct an expensive face-saving study to find a "scientific" explanation (2) to placate them.

Confidentiality of information in death certificates and other official documents is assured because custodians of these documents are sworn to secrecy. The code of conduct for official statisticians, developed by the International Statistical Institute (3), includes this obligation. It applies to epidemiologists who work with official documents such as birth and death certificates and census returns.

There is a "grey area" between these official

documents and other sources of information such as hospital records and health insurance claim forms. These records are among the most valuable varieties of health information; they have been essential to the discovery of many determinants of ill-health (4). However, political pressure aimed at protecting individual privacy can effectively deny access to them, and that would not be in the public interest. This ambiguous situation is among the motives to develop a code of ethics for epidemiologists.

If the code affirms confidentiality, access (in theory, anyway) may be more likely to be assured. In some countries, the political reality has been different, however: access has become more difficult, and has even been denied. Previously used sources that were integral components of record linkage systems sometimes have become inaccessible, even have been dismantled.

In Canada, reasoned argument by epidemiologists persuaded the committee drafting guidelines on ethics for the Medical Research Council to insert a clause explicitly recognizing the unique nature of epidemiological research: "... In cases such as epidemiological research where records of patients may be reviewed, the potential benefit and the degree of compromise of the patient's confidentiality must be carefully weighed by the (research ethics board)" (5). Nonetheless, hospital-based ethics review committees in Canada have still been known to obstruct access to medical records, interpreting their duties more rigidly than the Medical Research Council intended.

Who owns the data?

Another cause for concern has been freedom to use, discuss and publish all the information gathered in epidemiological studies. Questions have arisen about both raw and analysed data.

If an epidemiologist employed by an industrial corporation studies work-related illnesses of employees, the medical records (i.e., the actual pieces of paper) are the "property" of the corporation (although the individual records are confidential documents shared between each worker and the medical staff). Is the epidemiologist free to publish the results of analyses? Sometimes corporations have argued that the information belongs to them, the epidemiologist is employed by them, and only such information as they wish may be published. It is in the interests of the workers to know about hazardous working conditions and it is in the public interest for the facts to be widely known. Can the corporation prevent release of the findings? A similar question has arisen when a government has asserted that raw data and analysed results of publicly funded health research cannot be divulged wihout permission - which may be withheld, or made difficult and time-consuming to obtain.

The legal position regarding occupational and environmental health problems has been clarified in the United States and some other jurisdictions by "Right-to-know" legislation. The ethical position, i.e., the moral obligation of the epidemiologist to an employer, to the population studied, to a government or other funding agency, to the truth and to the public interest, is addressed in several draft codes of ethics for epidemiologists, described and discussed below. The moral stance in these draft codes of ethics is that data gathered in scientific studies should be subjected to critical peer review and should then enter the public domain. This applies in almost all scientific fields. Exceptions may be defence-related research and work that deals with trade secrets, e.g., genetic engineering techniques. Epidemiological research is not in either of these categories. But the exact chemical composition of substances used in patented processes is a trade secret, and it could be argued that therefore it is justifiable to withhold details if such compounds are imputed as a cause of occupational illness. Ethical and legal aspects of this problem require discussion as individual cases. No universal "rule" can be enunciated,

There is no moral or ethical justification for partial truth-telling, no public interest served, when governments or employers deny permission to publish an essential part of surveillance or research findings. If trade secrets are threatened, it is possible to find ways to compromise, e.g. by revealing generalities rather than specifics.

Presentation of research results

Epidemiologists are no more immune to dishonesty than scientists in other fields. Widely publicized instances of scientific fraud have drawn attention to the need for vigilance by peers, colleagues, editors of scientific journals (6). Pressure to produce and publish results is very high, especially among ambitious junior scientists, It can lead to unethical actions that have preoccupied biomedical science editors at several recent conferences (7). Fraud and plagiarism are rare; fictitious authorship is common. Common venial sins include duplicate and "salami" publication - slicing research reports into many thin pieces, called least publishable units or LPUs (8).

This pressure may also contribute to another problem that is not unique to epidemiology. This is the tendency for arguments about methods and procedures to be conducted in very public forums such as the correspondence columns of widely circulating general medical journals. Epidemiology depends upon balances among probabilities. When epidemiological evidence is used in law courts, the lawyers can impugn the credibility of their opponents by referring to the vituperative disputes that have festered in letters to editors of prestigious journals.

Codes and guidelines on ethics for epidemiologists

Following the example of other professional groups, several associations of epidemiologists have begun the task of developing ethics guidelines or codes of acceptable professional conduct for their members. The draft document prepared by Stolley and others (9) for the Society for Epidemiologic Research (SER) deals with conflict of interest. It addresses "ownership" of data, independence and integrity of investigators, publication of results; it is a brave but unenforcible statement, and it does not include logically presented arguments based on principles of biomedical ethics.

In Sweden, a committee of public health research workers (10) has compiled guidelines dealing with confidentiality, openness and access to information, responsibility for intervention, and storage and accessibility of data.

Cook, Beauchamp and Fayerweather (11) have produced for the Industrial Epidemiology Forum (IEF) in the USA, a draft Code of Ethics for Epidemiologists. This specifies obligations to research subjects (protecting welfare, obtaining informed consent, protecting pricavy, maintaining confidentiality, reviewing research protocols); obligations to society (avoiding conflict of interest, avoiding partiality); obligations to employers, funding agencies, etc (protecting privileged information); and obligations to colleagues (reporting methods and results, exposing unacceptable behavior or working conditions, communicating ethical requirements). An accompanying commentary sets the code in the context of ethical theory. This code is mainly intended for epidemiologists working in occupational settings, but many of its clauses apply more widely; some, however, do not acknowledge the variations in law, custom and culture that are to be found among the nations of the world. Like the much briefer SER draft, it is unenforcible.

The document that I am preparing (12) for the International Epidemiological Association (IEA) recognises the cultural, legal and regulatory diversity that make nonsense of ex cathedra statements about "right" and "wrong" courses of action. Basic concepts of autonomy that we take for granted are altogether different in some cultures. There are also differences in law and regulation among and even within nations, making it very difficult to establish a universally acceptable code of conduct for epidemiologists that is not so vague and general as to be useless. For example, in the United Kingdom, medical practitioners would be answerable in law (if not ethics) for the actions of non-medically qualified epidemiologists; in the United States, accountability is more widely diffused among health workers, regardless of their profession.

Is a code of conduct necessary for epidemiologists?

Pressure to write a code of conduct specifically for epidemiologists has come partly from non-medically qualified epidemiologists who have felt themselves professionally threatened, or asked to do things they find morally repugnant, for example by being prevented from releasing all the information that they have gathered. The proscription has usually come from employers, occasionally from government or other funding agencies.

A code of conduct, it is suggested, would strengthen the moral position of epidemiologists. Other arguments are that epidemiology has come of age as a discipline, and that like other health professions, psychologists, official statisticians, etc, epidemiologists ought to have a formal code of conduct. This would be a mark of professional maturity; and it would spell out the professional standards expected of epidemiologists.

Arguments against a formal code are that it creates rigidity in situations requiring flexibility of approach and response; that epidemiologists belong to professional groups who adhere to an existing code; that only confusion would result from yet another code, especially if its clauses differed from those of existing codes; on the other hand if they did not, what point would there be in producing yet another code? Further arguments are that a code would be unenforcible, and that it would be impossible to reconcile any code with the wide variations in national and local laws and regulations applying to such matters as protection of privacy.

Conclusion

There are some moral ambiguities in epidemiological practice and research. There is also great variation among the nations of the world in custom, tradition, law and regulation. The key work in discussing an ethical framework for epidemiology is flexibility. No rigid "rules" as set forth in a formal code of conduct can be responsive to such diversity.

When morally ambiguous situations arise, these require careful discussion that should involve all parties, including representatitives of public interest groups, health policy makers, management and labor, health care providers and users. It is often essential and always helpful to include also experts in ethical theory, and usually legal experts.

Afterthoughts

Impending events are likely to change our habitat, our way of life, our values - and therefore, our ethics, morality and our social and health policies.

There are ominous changes in planetary ecosystems (13). Global warming, ozone depletion and deteriorating environments threaten food security and water supplies. Collectively, these phenomena constitute the greatest ecological crisis since the last ice age; this is a real threat, unlike the theoretical threat of nuclear war.

Already there are millions of ecological refugees, crowded in periurban slums in third world cities, and altering the sociodemographic profile of industrial nations. Over the next fifty years, there will be many millions more. We can expect drastic changes in threats to individual and population health. We will be forced to put a higher priority on survival of human communities than on prolonging individual lives, which has been the main preoccupation of the medical profession in the past.

Very few people in any of the health professions seem willing even to think about these impending events. We must begin to discuss the health implications of global climate change, especially the ways in which this will force us to reappraise our priorities; and in the medical and other health professions, we must recognise our moral obligation to help guide human communities towards a more secure future.

References

1. Mortality Atlas of Canada, Volume 1: Cancer. Ottawa: Supply and Services Canada, 1980 (Cat. H49-6/1-1980); Mortality Atlas of Canada, Volume 2: General Mortality. Ottawa: Supply and Services Canada, 1980 (Cat. H49-6/2-1980).

2. Mao, Y., McCourt, C., Morrison, H., et al: Community-based mortality surveillance; the Maniwaki experience; investigation of excess mortality in a community. Can J Public Health 1984;75:429-433.

3. International Statistical Institute: Declaration on professional ethics. Internat Stat Rev, 1986;54: 227-242.

4. Last, J.M.: Epidemiology and health information, in Last J M (Ed), Maxcy-Rosenau Public Health and Preventive Medicine, 12th edition. Norwalk, CT: Appleton and Lange, 1986:9-74.

5. Medical Research Council of Canada: Guidelines on research involving human subjects. Ottawa: Medical Research Council, 1987.

6. Institute of Medicine Report on the responsible conduct of research in the health sciences. Clin Res, 1989;37:2:179-191.

7. Conferences held at the National Academy of Sciences, Washington, DC, in October 1988; "Ethics and Policy in Scientific Publishing" and in Chicago in May 1989; "First International Congress on Peer Review in Biomedical Publication".

8. Huth, E.J.: Irresponsible authorship and wasteful publication. Ann Int Med, 1986;104:257-259.

9. Stolley, P., Rothman, K., Shapiro, S., Stein, Z., Szklo, M.: Report of the Society for Epidemiologic Research Committee on Ethical Guidelines. May 1989.

10. Some ethical guidelines for public health research; deliberations of the Joint Committee for public health research. (English translation dated April 1989).

11. Cook, R., Beauchamp, T., Fayerweather, W.: Code of ethics for epidemiologists. Draft dated May 26, 1989.

12. Last, J.M.: Ethical guidelines for epidemiologists. December 1987.

13. Scientific American, September 1989: Managing planet earth (Special issue).

ETHICAL GUIDELINES AND CODES – CAN THEY BE UNIVERSALLY APPLICABLE IN A MULTI-CULTURAL WORLD?

Edward Keyserlingk

Efforts by international health-related agencies and associations to draft universally applicable ethics codes or guidelines encounter many obstacles and objections. The objection to be examined in this paper is that one or more of the provisions, or the whole set of guidelines, may not be acceptable to some member associations in view of the very different value systems, institutions, laws, social systems and social structures which prevail. That objection should be taken very seriously. Three standard or typical responses to that objection will be considered and rejected as inadequate. A fourth response, more sensitive to international multiculturalism and to the purpose of guidelines or codes, will then be proposed and examined.

Some make a distinction between a code of ethics and ethical guidelines, the former being allegedly more formal, fixed and rigid than the latter. That distinction may or may not be tenable, but even if it is, what follows is sufficiently general and fundamental to apply to both ethical guidelines or ethical codes.

This subject was selected for several related reasons. First of all, this paper is meant to be at least a partial and tentative answer to one of the questions addressed in this section, "Should ethical standards be regarded as matters of cultural customs, or universally applied?" Secondly, the International Epidemiological Association (IEA) is in the process of formulating a set of ethical guidelines. There has been some discussion and debate in the Association about those guidelines in view of cultural differences between member associations, and it is hoped that what follows will prove to be a useful contribution to that debate and to similar debates in other health-related associations. Thirdly, the role of ethics in multi-cultural contexts is one which has been largely neglected to this point, and one which is of increasing interest. While my direct focus will be on ethical guidelines or codes, I hope my remarks will be applicable beyond just the making of guidelines, and beyond just the context of epidemiology.

It is arguable that the drafters of professional codes of ethics and ethical guidelines in the area of health care and research over the past many years and still today, tend to implicitly or explicitly adopt one of three responses to the multicultural factor. Each of them in effect ascribes a different moral weight to cultural considerations.

1. Some associations or agencies are very aware of the multi-cultural reality, and at least partly for that reason they leave the code's provisions at a very high level of abstraction. The result: codes which are correspondingly remote and utopian, but (at least in the view of their drafters) culturally non-offensive.

2. A second option by way of response to the multi-cultural factor is to more or less ignore that perspective, in which case the dominant cultural and political element in the code-writing committee will tend (often quite unconsciously) to impose its own culture-conditioned values, principles and practices as the normative standards. For the most part the dominant cultural and political orientation of these committees has been and continues to be, western. This second approach tends to give little or no serious attention to debate or refinement in the light of the experience and insights of other cultures and traditions.

3. A third approach and response gives a great deal of weight to the multi-cultural reality of member associations, so much so that it leads to abandoning efforts to formulate a universally applicable set of ethical guidelines. It is left to each member association in different parts of the world to produce its own code or guidelines reflecting the distinct values, culture, institutions and practices of its particular society. Those of this view, conclude that it is unrealistic and intrusive to do otherwise.

But what makes all three of those options inadequate is that they either give the multicultural factor too little weight or too much weight. In both cases, it is assumed that there can be no real meeting of minds across cultures to the benefit of everyone, no space given for cultural and ethical variations, which leads to one of three results: excessive ethical generality which achieves little for anyone; ethical/cultural domination by one perspective over all the others, or a defeatist paralysis which leaves intact and undisturbed the ethical/cultural walls between societies.

The next step is to outline the ingredients of what could be called a fourth option, one which could be sensitive to many traditions and cultures and universally applicable yet provide an effective code of ethics or set of ethical guidelines. There are, it could be argued, six such ingredients in this fourth option:

1. Though compromise should be resisted on what are finally determined and agreed upon to be the ethical essentials of such a code of ethics, input into its formulation should be invited and facilitated from the start of deliberations from a representative number of associations and cultures comprising the membership. The goal should not be to water down the provisions or find the lowest ethical common denominator. Rather the purpose of this wide multicultural involvement would be twofold. First of all, in order to capture within the guidelines for the benefit of epidemiologists and publics everywhere the valuable moral insights and experience of many societies in the struggle against disease and for the protection of persons and populations. Secondly, to allow for as much adaptation as possible to those different traditions, customs, value systems and social structures.

2. The process should start by seeking agreement upon a set of general principles and guidelines, though only as a first step towards addressing more specific issues and implications. This first step involves not only seeking agreement upon the normative values, principles and interests, but also how they should be ranked and balanced in various circumstances, and even more fundamentally and before that, how these values should be understood, described and situated given the multi-cultural perspective.

We should pause and comment on these first two aspects of this option. The difficulties involved in attempting to bridge the vast cultural gaps between western concepts of person and morality, and those of many other non-western societies should not be underestimated. But nor should we underestimate the potential rewards of even partial success in such bridging efforts. Examples of the cultural gaps and their relevance for efforts to construct universally applicable ethical guidelines are easily uncovered. One major constellation of values in western culture is that of "individualism", which underlies western interpretations of freedom, liberty, autonomy and rights. Codes of ethics or ethical guidelines largely formulated by or influenced by westerners consistently give a central place to personal autonomy, from which flow a variety of rights such as informed consent, inviolability, privacy and confidentiality. The draft guidelines of the IEA are no exception.

For western biomedicine (as in most other areas of western society), the "individual" has distinct priority over society, is culturally distinct from society and even in conflict with it (1). This is particularly the case in North America. Society tends to be based more on atomism than on holism (2), leading to relationships which are more contractual than organic. That in turn, suggests moral codes of "rights" rather than "duties". The person in the European Protestant tradition tends to be seen in isolation from his social position, role and context, whereas in many other traditions and societies, persons are not defined separately from the context, but in varying degrees in socially relative ways. This western concept of self has been described as identified not with the physical body, but with the conscious self, the seat of control (2). Consistent with this concept is the prevailing view that to be socially determined is to be trapped, weak and limited. Foucault and others have pointed out how not only the body has been objectified, but the self as well, autonomous, self-determining, not determined by its values, traditions or relations with others (4).

> Gordon (1) wrote that the ideal moden entity:
>
> "...is as free of traces of social and cultural determination as possible. It strives to be its own author, consciously choosing its path, able to disengage itself and step back and judge rationally what it will be, where it will go. Self control by the modern entity is potentially unlimited".
>
> Kirmayer (5) gave a similar description of the western concept:
>
> "...a rational agent which occupies a space within the body, which itself dwells within the social world. The self has goals that are distinct from, and in many cases in conflict with, the goals of others who occupy the social world outside. The value of the person lies in his strength or will which is defined always in opposition to the other - whether that other be society, nature or the body itself. The person is identical with that rational agency that establishes its unique worth by promoting its own goals over those of others. The potential divisiveness of this individualism and rational self-interest is held in check by appeals to moral obligation.

Because western morality considers the individual a core value, it is dedicated to defending the individual's sovereignty, ensuring freedom from interference, and promoting equal treatment and opportunity for development. All of this is typically expressed in a language of rights. The freedom sought is absolute and universal. Little attention or support is directed to society in western morality, and little focus on the ethics of responsibility, responding to needs and not just to rights.

Against that background it is hardly surprising that the prevailing ideal models of social relationships in western biomedicine are those resulting from contracts consented to by autonomous individuals. The prevailing language of bioethics in the west is a rights language, undoubtedly in many respects contributed to by patients finding themselves increasingly in impersonal institutional settings treated by a host of nameless specialists. The emphasis is on protecting patient autonomy against encroachment and paternalism, not on rights to community, caring or kindness (6, 7).

The emphasis on contracts between informed partners may well be a needed corrective to years of medical domination; they may also be seen as a continuing rebellion against the need by individuals for society, for nurturing, for dependence (1).

That other non-western societies tend to understand and situate persons very differently is no longer a novel observation. Consider Japan for example. Love (for example between mother and the child) comes from belonging more than from striving, not so much from controlling as from fitting in. As Kirmayer notes, a result is that the sense of opposition between the self and others is more muted (4, 5). Autonomous acts are much less prized than is social connectedness.

In Japan, as in many other societies, it is the family unit more than the individual which is the locus of decisions. In the west we tend to assume that it is the patient or the research subject who makes decisions, the issue being therefore not so much who makes the decision, but what kind of information and capacity they need to make it. But in fact such decisions in more "traditional" societies tend to be made in a group context, and matters of status, age, rank and sex will often be crucially important elements. An example implicating epidemiology is that of family planning programs in Indonesia, a major government and health clinic priority. The program established was technically excellent, but only moderately successful. The rate of acceptance for family planning remained low. One of the major reasons for that appears to be that it was based upon the erroneous assumption that it was the woman herself who made that decision (8). As a result, all the education and propaganda efforts were directed exclusively to the wives. In fact their views on that subject and others were the least important in the family. The major decisions tend to be made by the husband, and on matters such as children and grandchildren the views of grandparents are also considered most important.

Similar evidence has long been available in many other societies about the centrality of the social context and the family unit, whether they be Inuits in the north or Greek immigrants in Montreal.

In view of the wide cultural gap between western and more traditional societies on such a fundamental matter, what should be done regarding universally applicable ethical guidelines? What precedes may seem to be a compelling argument for leaving it to each society to formulate its own code, its own ethical guidelines. But that would be regrettable and premature. In fact, we have not even begun to seriously try to bridge the conceptual and ethical gap, to seek common denominators while respecting cultural/social differences, at least not regarding morality and moral obligations. At least three good reasons exist for making the effort.

First of all, great strides have been made at the level of health program development and delivery by international agencies in moderating western attitudes of superiority. It used to be more typical than it is for international public health programs to assume that if the program was scientifically sound, the people in the target society would enthusiastically embrace it and cooperate. That assumption in turn was based on the conviction that western civilization was so superior to technologically less complex societies that people in "less fortunate" countries would love to adopt our ways (8). Happily today, in the face of many years of evidence that scientific medicine is not automatically welcomed everywhere, and that the cultural differences do count, that western ethnocentricity is much less evident.

But what needs to be done now is to go one big step further and subject western ethnocentricity, at the level of moral concepts and moral obligations, to the same critical analysis already well underway at the clinical and program level.

A second reason why we must make the attempt is that we in the west are increasingly aware of the limits of our almost exclusive reliance on a rights-based bioethics, which focuses too exclusively on individual autonomy to the exclusion of human needs, the interdependence between persons and society, and decision making as a reflection of social values and group benefit. If western biomedicine and bioethics (including codes of ethics) are ever to recover a more holistic stance, it will surely be in large part the result of serious dialogue and interaction with members of societies which have retained a fuller concept of what it is to be persons.

Does it follow then that universal ethical guidelines or codes should jettison the moral principles and rules central to the existing codes? Not necessarily. But insofar as they are intended to be international they do need broadening and they do need at least in some respects a new language, and they do need more "variations on the themes". For example, serious reflection and cross-cultural dialogue may well reveal that the (Kantian) moral principle of "respect for persons" has strong roots or equivalents in societies other than western, but if so, "person" cannot be any longer the individual atom distinct from society and culture, but person in its full social and cultural context.

3. The long-range goal of the code formulation process should be more than just a set of general guidelines based on general principles, but should also provide specific and more detailed directions on a variety of issues arising, in this case, in the practice of epidemiology. Given the increasing complexity of the issues and the many factors to be balanced and integrated, general principles and guidelines alone are decreasingly helpful and normative. The mere assertion and listing of the fundamental normative principles, and the basic rights and duties derived from them is in itself difficult and challenging, especially in a multicultural context. But the next and indispensable stage must be that of ranking them, that is, determining the scope of each of them when they compete and conflict in a variety of contexts and issues.

An example of such a specific issue is that of the control of, access to and sharing of sensitive epidemiological data. A set of internationally applicable ethical guidelines would both describe and prescribe data collection and storage precautions which could ensure the access required for the protection of public health officials without unduly risking confidentiality. Whether such more detailed provisions should be attached to the general guidelines as integral parts, or produced subsequently and on an on-going basis is another matter.

4. Both the general and the more specific guidelines should be envisaged and promulgated as normative and not just elective goals for all member associations.

There is a compelling reason why that is almost self-evident, at least about some issues. Assume for example that it is decided to include some specific guidelines on the screening, research and treatment of infections diseases. Insofar as those provisions are applicable to AIDS/HIV, given international travel and immigration we do not have the luxury of leaving it to each country to decide whether and how to deal with it. As an international epidemic AIDS/HIV requires coordinated and consistent approaches.

At a more fundamental level, the _purpose_ of codes of ethics or ethical guidelines must be grappled with. There are two major options in this regard. For some, codes of ethics only mirror the positive morality of the members of the profession or discipline involved. There is little doubt that this is what in fact some codes do, though it is not the same as concluding that this is all they should do. One commentator writes for example, that modern codes

> "...can reasonably be expected to reflect the basic ethical views of the organizations that endorsed them. In fact it might be argued that documents that are the product of practitioners rather than theoreticians reflect even more accurately the ethical stance of the group than do more systematic efforts at developing theories of medical ethics" (9).

That may be generally true of codes of ethics in recent times, but it was certainly not the case with earlier codes inspired by exemplars of practice such as Hippocrates, Percival, Maimonides and many others. Those oaths and statements were looked up to as challenges, as examples of excellence rather than just reflections of a minimum morality, or the lowest common denominator. There is then a second option regarding the purpose of codes and ethical guidelines, which looks to them as having universal normative validity, as challenges to do better, to reform and improve conduct, customs, laws and institutions which fall below the established mark. It is arguable that to conclude otherwise would be to betray the letter and spirit of the many U.N. and W.H.O. health and research related codes and constitutions. For the most part they were responses to perceived immoralities and injustices, challenges and injunctions to do better, not just reflections of prevailing practices. They were and are meant to be universally applied and they provide no exceptions for particular cultures or societies. They must now be brought a big step forward by revising them in the direction of more sensitivity to international and national multi-culturalism, but there can be no doubt that they were meant to be (and rightly so) normative rather than just descriptive.

A recent example of how the process of code writing can take a code and a profession a few steps closer to excellence can be seen in the evolution of the American Medical Association's position on the treatment of patients with AIDS. In its 1986 statement it singled out AIDS as a reason for refusing to treat a person, but in a 1987 statement it in effect acknowledged the right to treatment of patients with AIDS. What appears to have led to the change was the realization that the earlier position was inconsistent with its stance on professional obligations as expressed in its code of ethics and elsewhere (10).

5. It is arguable that a universally applicable code of ethics or set of guidelines should give some attention to "macro-ethical" and not just "micro-ethical" matters. Epidemiologists, after all, have as one of their professional mandates that of uncovering factors which influence health related states or events, in order to enhance the health of populations and individuals.

That "population-based" aspect of epidemiology would seem to justify and even oblige that some serious attention be given to economic, environmental, political, institutional and structural perspectives. For example, the evidence mounts that the widespread, excessive and often uncontrolled use of pesticides in many developing countries is causing health problems of major proportions. Serious inequities with severe health realted effects, not least of them famine, are often built into the social and political fabric of many countries.

It is not of course a novel proposal that epidemiologists should concern themselves with these "macro" issues. But if that is so, then it seems to follow that their obligations in that regard should also be reflected in their internationally applicable code of ethics.

Two cautions are, however, in order. One has to do with the cultural sensitivity issue already referred to. One of the inhibitions inevitably imposed by being sensitive to the cultures and societies of others is that it becomes less obvious when a problem is a real, objective evil (by everyone's standards) which merits attention and righteous indignation, and when on the other hand, it is an evil only when seen through the subjective eyes of those from another culture. Famines brought on by the neglect, abuse and infighting of a country's leaders would seem to fall readily into the first category. Both locals and outsiders of other cultures are likely to agree. For many other problems it is less evident. The issue of moral relativity inevitably must be faced and dealt with in any effort to produce codes of ethics for multi-cultural contexts.

However behind such neglect and cruelty we <u>may</u> sometimes find a more fundamental or contributing wrong perpetrated by a more developed western country which has ignored the plight and requests of the poorer country or has for example intervened in its markets or politics in such a way that tribal warfare and famine was inevitable.

A second caution has to do with the ever-present danger of forcing non-medical concerns into the medical model by assuming that epidemiologists have the training and mandate to attack all problems in the economic, political and other areas (11). But while that danger is real it would be less so if it were to be clearly stated and understood that epidemiologists must at the macro-level work closely with those of many other disciplines - anthropologists, economists, ethicists, lawyers, etc.

6. A last ingredient of this option I am proposing begins with the reminder that the moral injunctions of such a code should be seen as long term <u>goals,</u> not realizable everywhere right away or in the near future.

Many countries are not well endowed with the

experienced people, finances or institutions needed to establish for instance review boards to assure valid research. In my view, when an international association decides to formulate a set of normative ethical guidelines for all its member associations, the association itself incurs a moral obligation to assist its members and branches in the task of establishing or adapting structures and resources to give effect to those guidelines. Otherwise it is setting impossible goals, and impossible goals cannot be ethical goals.

References

1. Gordon, D.R.: Tenacious Assumptions in Western Medicine, in Lock, M., and Gordon, D.R. (eds.) Biomedicine Examined. Kluwer, 1988.

2. Dumont, L.: Homo Hierarchicus. London: Paladin, 1970.

3. Geertz, C.: On the nature of anthropological understanding. In: Annual Editions in Anthropology. Guilford, Conn.: Duskin, 1977.

4. Foucault, M.: The order of things - the archeology of the human sciences. New York: Vintage, 1973.

5. Kirmayer, L.J.: Mind and body as metaphor: Hidden values in biomedicine, in Lock, M., and Gordon, D.R. (eds.) Biomedicine Examined. Kluwer, 1988.

6. Fox, R.C., and Swazey, J.P.: Medical morality is not bioethics - medical ethics in China and the United States. Perspectives in Biology and Medicine 1984;27:336-360.

7. Zaner, R.: Chance and morality: The dialysis phenomenon, in Kestenbaum, V. (ed.). The Humanity of the Ill. Knoxville, U. of Tenn. Press, 1982.

8. Foster, G.M., and Anderson, B.G.: Medical Anthropology. New York: J. Wiley, 1978.

9. Veatch, R.M.: Codes of medical ethics: Ethical analysis, in Reich, W., and Walters, L. (eds.) Encyclopedia of Bioethics (Vol.1). New York: Free Press, 1988.

10. Freedman, B.: Health professionals, codes and the right to refuse to treat HIV-infectious patients.

Hastings Center Report 1988:18:20-25.

11. Goodman, L.E., and Goodman, M.J.: Prevention, how misuse of a concept undercuts its worth. Hastings Center Report 1986;16:26-38.

ETHICAL ASPECTS ON EPIDEMIOLOGICAL RESEARCH

Peter Allebeck

There is no clear-cut boundary between epidemiological and other types of biomedical research, and the basic ethical principles for epidemiological research are not distinct from those of research ethics in general. There are, however, some characteristics of epidemiological research which in many cases require special ethical considerations. Basing myself on these special characteristics, I will discuss some ethical aspects on epidemiological research, and focus on the researchers responsibility in maintaining a good ethical conduct. If the scientific community does not take the responsibility for maintaining high ethical standards, and work along the lines suggested in the paper by John M Last, I think it will be difficult to prevent further restrictions of legal and administrative nature on epidemiological research (1).

Characteristics of epidemiological research

What are the special characteristics of epidemiological research compared to other types of biomedical research? A Swedish working party involved in ethics in epidemiology tentatively defined three characteristics, of which at least one generally should be present in order that a given project should be included under the broad heading of epidemiological research:

1. Number of persons involved in the study. This may be an important feature of an epidemiological study, particularly when large population based registers are being used. I should point out that many epidemiological studies are not based on large numbers of persons investigated, and that the population based character of a study is more a question of how the subjects have been selected and for what purpose rather than the number in itself. But in many cases the numbers are important.

2. The research is often of a non-experimental or observational nature. We can not deliberately expose persons to different levels of smoking, alcohol consumption, environmental hazards, etc, or randomize persons into different occupations in order to elucidate health risks. What we can do is to make use of the variability created by differences in genetic setup, behaviour, occupation, life style, etc, in different groups. By using methods for observation of exposure and outcome, and by using adequate methods of analysis, hypotheses can be tested more or less as validly as in experimental studies.

3. The researcher is usually not involved in a doctor-patient relation. One obvious reason is that the subjects are often not patients but healthy persons. When patients are subjects of study in an epidemiological investigation, the researcher is usually someone else than the treating physician. And the interviews are often performed by special interviewers who are not part of the health care team.

Since a large part of epidemiological research is in fact public health research, I would like to point out another distinction, and that is that towards public health in itself, its policy-making, planning and administration. The distinction between public health research and public health policy may seem obvious, but there are several examples from Sweden and Stockholm in which disputes over general public health related matters have been turned into matters of research ethics. Without going into details here, I can think of two projects that were submitted to the research ethics committee at the Karolinska Institute. One concerned the introduction of the total artificial heart, the other concerned a large community survey in Stockholm County. There was criticism and dispute regarding these projects in general; the way they were planned, how decisions were taken how the resources were allocated etc. There were also specific aspects of research ethics, but the way the policy making bodies referred the matters to the research ethics committee, was as I see it a way to avoid a serious debate on key issues at the appropriate level. The system for ethical review of research projects should not be used for other purposes in the absence of proper fora for debate on ethical issues in public health.

Ethical problems related to specific characteristics

What are the specific research ethical problems related to the three characteristics of epidemiological research enumerated above?

1. The number of subjects involved in a study should generally not in itself have special ethical implications. However, since large scale epidemiological studies imply large data bases with much data on many persons, we often have to face the ethical concerns raised regarding comprehensive data bases. Concern has been expressed as to how data are being stored and handled, for what purposes they might be used, and possible risk of misuse, e.g. that unauthorized persons should get access to the data base and retrieve delicate information on individuals.

As scientists we know that in these expressed concerns there is often a confounding with administrative data bases. We know that epidemiologists are not interested in data on individuals but data on groups, and that access to computerized data generally is much more difficult than paper based records and that the risk of inappropriate use is minimal compared to many other types of data handling. Nevertheless, the concern has to be taken seriously, and the scientific community should take all steps to ensure confidentiality of personal data, security in the storing and handling of data and guarantee that data collected for research purpose are not used for other purposes (2,3). The principal investigator has an important task in informing the public, policy-makers and of course the subjects involved about how these basic ethical requirements are being met, and, what might be even more important the aims and objectives of any research project. Only in this way can we prevent that legislators and policy-makers strongly restrict - if not make totally impossible - the use of computerized health related data bases for research purposes.

2. Regarding the observational versus experimental research design, it is clear that the declaration of Helsinki was elaborated to regulate biomedical experiments on human beings, and the history of this declaration goes back to the atrocities performed during Nazi Germany. This means that epidemiological methods for enquiring about exposures and outcomes are not really covered by the Helsinki declaration (4).

Instruments of observational research

The instruments of observational research are for example interviews and questionnaires. It is clear that interviews and questionnaires on personal matters may be just as controversial and threatening to the integrity of the individual as many experimental manipulations. Not long ago, it was rare that an interview study was submitted to a research ethics committee. The attitude has now changed, and there is a consensus in most countries that studies based on questionnaires or interviews should be submitted to a research ethics committee for assessment, including the protocols.

Sometimes instruments for observation are obtained from records and data bases not primarily set up for research purposes. In occupational epidemiology employment rolls are often used for information on exposure to a certain occupation. Sometimes very specific data on duration and type of occupational exposure can be obtained. Data from population and housing censuses are used to determine exposure to environmental hazards, such as radon in the ground and proximity to high energy electric cables, to mention a few ongoing projects. Many of these data are administrative data, basically collected for other purposes than research. To what extent and by which procedures these can be used for research purposes is a matter of judgment, and a research ethics committee has to take a decision in each individual case. In many cases data collected for a specific purpose can not be used for other purposes. But the examples above can hardly be considered controversial, and many similar examples can be found

(3,5).

Intervention responsibility

3. In epidemiological research there is usually no direct doctor-patient relation between the researcher and those who are subjects of study. The question of intervention responsibility may therefore be slightly more complicated than in clinical research. Different levels of intervention can be conceived. The most obvious example is that of an epidemiological survey with a personal interview and some kind of physical examination. In this situation it is clear that any health problem detected must be taken care of in some way, usually by referral to appropriate health services. In this way the investigation can also be of advantage to the individual. It is a service we can offer in exchange of the subjects' participation in the project.

But take the example where HIV is being tested for. The researcher may only be interested in prevalence data and often prefers to do anonymous testing. But the subject may want to know the result, and should have the right to, if blood is drawn. How should this be arranged? Who should communicate the results? Who should be responsible for the proper handling of the case? What about notification to public health authorities if there is such a regulation? These are just some questions of many that may have to be dealth with. They illustrate the importance of well defining in advance the level of intervention and the procedures by which health care measures should be undertaken. This should also be explained clearly in the information to the participants.

Another type of intervention problem is when plasma or any other substance is being stored, a rather common procedure in longitudinal studies. It happens that a previously unknown disease marker is discovered and identified in individuals included in the study. Scrutiny of records may also reveal health problems. Should the subjects be informed about such findings? No general answer can be given. A research ethics committee may have to be consulted. In the working party previously mentioned we said that if information appears that may be of importance for the life and health of the subjects, they should be informed and appropriate action taken. But it is hardly ethical to inform about vaguely known possible risk factors for disease just for the sake of giving full and honest information.

The third aspect of intervention i would like to mention is that connected with screening for disease in programmes for secondary prevention. We can take the example of mammographic screening for early detection of breast cancer. A number of population based trials have been performed to assess whether mammographic screening reduces the mortality in breast cancer. The overall results have indicated a slight but statistically significant reduction in breast cancer mortality among those who have undergone the screening programme. The classical ethical problems regarding the risks of the screening programme, and the worry and anguish among those who have to come back for further assessment, versus the benefit of reduced mortality and morbidity in breast cancer, have been amply discussed (6,7). But very little has been discussed about different possible levels of intervention on those who are invited to the programme. Is it ethical to call thousands, millions of women to a screening programme in which they are only put in front of a camera to detect a possible breast cancer. How about those who smoke 10-20 cigarettes a day? How about those with excessive alcohol consumption and perhaps small children? Can we just leave these other risk groups, giving them the knowledge that at least they do not have breast cancer - at least not right now. On 50 year old men all kinds of intervention programmes have been tried and evaluated. I think we need a scientific and ethical debate on what types of intervention programmes should be offered to 50 year old women, besides the pure radiological screening (8).

Conclusion

To conclude, there is no clear-cut boundary between epidemiological and other types of biomedical research. Neither are the general ethical issues of epidemiological research very different from those of research ethics in general. There are some characteristics of epidemiological research who call for special ethical considerations, particularly since these problems are not covered by the declaration of Helsinki. Researchers in epidemiology and public health have an important task in informing the public and policy-makers about these matters, thereby preventing that further restrictions by ignorance will be imposed on this type of research.

References

1. Rothman, K.J.: The rise and fall of epidemiology 1950-2000 A.D. N Engl J Med 1981;304:600-602.

2. Gordis, L., Gold, E., Seltser, R.: Privacy protection and medical research: A challenge and a responsibility. Am J Epidemiol 1977;105:163-168.

3. Lako, C.J.: Privacy protection and population-based health research. Soc Sci Med 1986;23:293-295.

4. Soskolne, C.: Epidemiology: Questions of science, ethics, morality and law. Am J Epidemiol 1989;129:1-18.

5. Gordis, L., Gold, E.: Privacy, confidentiality and the use of medical records in research. Science 1980;207:153-156.

6. Skrabanek, P.: False premises and false promises of breast cancer screening. Lancet 1985;2:316-19.

7. Eddy, DM., McGivney, W.: The value of mammographic screening in women under age 50 years. J Am Med Ass 1988;259:1512-1519.

8. Brett, AS.: Ethical issues in risk factor intervention. Am J Med 1984;76:557-561.

ETHICAL AND LEGAL PROBLEMS IN RESEARCHER'S ACCESS TO DATA STORES

Jochanan Benbassat
Micha Levy

Epidemiologic research, similarly to clinical research in general, should be based on the vaules "do no harm" and "respect people's integrity". "Do no harm" means that clinical experiments may not compromise the health of the test subject; "Respect people's integrity" is the basis of the requirement of a competent, free and informed consent (1,2).

For prospective clinical experiments, these two values have been translated into defined rules and regulations. However, there are no clear-cut provisions pertaining to the retrospective use of stored data, such as medical records. Thus, it is uncertain, whether retrospective surveys of medical records or reexamination of stored material, such as frozen samples of sera, should be conditional on the patients' informed consent.

Informed consent is not an ethical requirement only, but also a legal prerequisite. During the last 20 years there has been a tendency in many countries to legislate for the protection of privacy, particularly in the field on computerized data. In Israel the legal definition of "Infringement of Privacy" includes "infringing on a duty of secrecy laid down by express or implicit agreement in respect of a person's private affairs; using or passing on to another information on a person's private affairs otherwise than for the purpose for which it was given" (3). The implication of this legislation is that informed consent should be a prerequisite for research based on information compiled for other purposes, such as medical records or other data, which were not initially meant to serve for medical purposes.

The ethical principle of "respect people" and the legal restriction of use of stored data raise the following questions regarding retrospective epidemiologic surveys: (a) Are studies of medical records or of stored material, such as frozen samples of sera or paraffin blocks of biopsies tissue, permissible without the informed consent of the patient? (b) if so - should the medical archives in hospitals be made available to anybody engaged in bona fide research? (c) Would the situation be different if every patient admitted to hospital was requested to waive his right of confidentiality of health related information for purposes of research? and (d) May files compiled with the patient's consent by one researcher be transferred to another one or linked to other files of stored data, whether medical or not?

For many, these questions may seem to be a needless and dogmatic complication of the issue. After all, what could be the ethical problems of the following hypothetial research proposal:

> A retrospective study of all cases with Polymyositis - Dermatomyositis (PM-DM) is performed by reviewing the records of all hospitals in Israel. The anticipated total number of cases with PM-DM in the last 30 years does not exceed 100. Should these patients be asked to consent to such a study? Should the relatives of the deceased patients be contacted for consent?

What possible harm or disrespect can be inflicted to patients with PM-DM by reviewing their charts or even reexamining their biopsies? None of course. Yet, other retrospective research proposals may be more problematic:

In 1976 informed consent is obtained from a number of subjects to a study designed to investigate the incidence of Hepatitis B antigen (HBag). After testing for HBag, the sera are frozen and stored. Can these sera be tested in 1985 for antibodies to HIV without obtaining the consent of the subjects? Can these sera be given to another researcher for this purpose? Would this researcher be free to contact some or all test subjects and ask them about their sexual preferences?

A retrospective study is designed to test the hypothesis that women with a certain blood group miscarry more often. Could this hypothesis be tested by a survey of hospital charts? Is the compilation of a list of women who aborted permissible? Can they be contacted and asked to participate in a study related to abortion?

A prospective longitudinal study is started in 1963 aimed at defining maternal perinatal risk indicators regarding the offspring. At that time no informed consent is obtained. However the intention of the researcher, at the time, is to restrict the study to the perinatal period. Can the compiled file be transferred to somebody else? Could this same file be used for follow-up of the children through their adolescence? Can the data be linked to police records in order to look for predictive indicators of delinquency without the consent of the subjects?

The simplest way to deal with the ethical and legal problems arising from retrospective epidemiologic surveys would be to impose a requirement of informed consent from all subjects participating in retrospective surveys. However, a requirement of informed consent from a large number of patients before examining their records would preclude the performance of most retrospecive and prospective clinical studies (4-7). Even when feasible, i.e., even when all patients whose charts should be surveyed are alive and available, it is still uncertain how energetically informed consent may be sought without harassment of the subject, considering the necessity to obtain a maximal response rate (8).

Some authors (4) have considered the possibility of a general consent obtained from patients on admission to hospital to use their charts for future research purposes with the understanding that the patients will not be identified and their privacy will be safeguarded. Such a general consent is legally worthless; furthermore, it is not an acceptable ethical substitute for informed consent. "Informed" consent can only be given by a subject after he has received an explanation of the purposes of the planned research, and after he has been offered the option to decline. Some subjects for example, may not want to participate in a research aiming to identify racial differences in intelligence. Moreover, the subject must be told the reasons for his selection; the research procedures must be explained; the expected duration of his participation must be stated; the subject must be warned about possible discomforts and risks; he must be given a description of the benefits for others; and measures to ensure confidentiality must be explained (2). Obviously, therefore, we are faced with the choice of forgoing the rule of informed consent, and discontinuing epidemiologic research.

Discontinuation of epidemiologic research will affect adversely clinical practice. As pointed out by Sackett et al, "the important acts we carry out as clinicians require the particularization, to the individual patient, of our prior experiences (both as individual clinicians and collectivey) with groups of similar patients" (8). The care of individual patients necessitates the rational application of the principles of population epidemiology. Consequently, we must seek ways to exempt investigators involved in retrospective studies of medical records or of stored material (e.g., frozen samples of sera or paraffin blocks of biopsies tissue) from obtaining the patients' informed consent, and still abide by the principles "do no harm" and "respect people's integrity".

There are exceptional cases in which it is ethically permissible to forgo informed consent. For example, the US National Commission for the Protection of Human subjects of Biomedical and Behavioral Research (9) has recommended that informed consent is unnecessary, when (1) the subject's interests are determined to be adequately protected.... and the importance of the research justifies such invasion of the subject's privacy. (b) The use or disclosure of the information does not violate any limitations under which the record or information was collected, and (c) The disclosed information might not significantly change the way in which the individual is perceived by self, family, social group, employer, and should not expose the individual to liability for criminal or other action.

We suggest to amend the Law for Protection of Privacy in Israel along these recommendaions (9). Retrospective studies involving medical records, records compiled for other purposes, reexamination of stored biological material, transfer of files compiled with the patient's consent by one researcher to another, or linkage among records from various sources, should be permitted even without informed consent, subject to approval by "Institutional Review Boards (IRBs). In such cases IRBs should be aware of their additional resposibility to protect patients from unwarranted discomfort, unnecessary invasion of privacy and from involuntary participation in research to which they might object because of values or ideology.

We propose that the following conditions should be fulfilled prior to exempting an investigator from obtaining an informed consent from the subjects participating in epidemiologic studies: (a) The IRB members should agree on the merit of the research project and on the ability of the investigator to carry it out. (b) An assurance should be provided by the investigator that the subject's identity will be kept in confidence, and that the data will be used only for scientific purposes. (c) Contacts with the patient during the study (if any) will not result in an unacceptable unpleasantness, and considering the prevailing local cultural trends, it is unlikely that the patient would object to the goals of the research, and (d) The research does not violate the patient's right for privacy, e.g., linkage with stored "sensitive" data from other resources. To this end, the term "right for privacy" will have to be redefined.

According to these criteria, projects similar to those presented in example 1 should be permissible even in the absence of the patients' consent. Such a research does not impinge on the patients' privacy and does not raise the danger of litigation. It seems that the Israeli Protection of Privacy Law considered such a contingency in stating that "No right to bring a civil or criminal action under this Law shall accrue through an infringement of no real significance" (3). However, unlike example 1, example 2 presents a situation in which it is conceivable that the patients will not be indifferent to the research project and that at least some of them may not agree with its goals. The possibility that some of them may refuse to participate in such a study makes informed consent mandatory.

Examples 3 and 4 illustrate the "gray zone" within which IRBs should exercise their judgement. Within certain constraints, parts of these studies may be permitted, subject to strict adherence to the deletion of any personal identification parameters. It may be argued, that in each of these situations the mere approach of the patient in order to obtain his informed consent may result in an unacceptable unpleasantness. Both involve invasion into a domain considered personal by current social norms. In each case the IRB will have to decide the degree to which the approach of the patients is an invasion of privacy, which may in itself result in anguish, and rule accordingly. We believe that cross-linkage with police records as proposed in example 4 should not be permitted under any circumstances.

References

1. Dubcan, A.S., Dunstan, G.R., Wilburn, R.B.: Dictionary of medical ethics. London, Darton, Longman and Todd. 2nd ed, 1981.

2. Levine, R.J.: Ethics and regulations of clinical research. 2 ed. Urban and Schartzenberg, Baltimore, 1986.

3. Laws of the State of Israel. Protection of Privacy Law. 5741 - 1981. Vol 35, p.136, Sections 2(7) and 2(9).

4. Appelbaum, P.S., Roth, L.H., Detre, T.: Researchers' access to patients' records. An analysis of the ethical problems. Clinical Research, 1984;33:-399-403.

5. Waters, W.E.: Ethics and epidemiological research. Intern J Epidemiol, 1985;14:48-51.

6. Rothman, K.J.: The rise and fall of epidemiology. N Engl J Med, 1981;304:600.

7. Holder, A.R., Levine, R,J.: Informed consent for research on specimens obtained at autopsy or surgery: a case study in the overprotection of

human subjects. Clin Res, 24:68-77 (1976).

8. Sackett, D.L., Haynes, R.B., Tugwell, P.: Clinical epidemiology. Little Brown Co, Boston (1985).

9. The National Commission for the Protection of Human subjects of Biomedical and Behavioral Research: Institutional Review Boards: Report and Recommendations. DHEW Publication No. (OS) 78-0008, Appendix, DHEW Publication No.(OS)78-0009, Washington, 1978.

The paper is based on an article published in IRB: A review of Human Subjects Research, May/June 1988.

ETHICAL PROBLEMS IN EPIDEMIOLOGICAL RESEARCH: DISCUSSION

Göran Hermerén

Introduction

Let me begin by comparing two relatively simple cases. Let us first suppose that a person has a dog which is discovered to have an incurable cancer. Let us moreover suppose that the dog is in constant pain. In that case it would be unfair against the dog, in the view of most people, not to take it to the vet and ask him to give it a painless death. Those who did not do so would be accused of egoism and of not putting the dog's best interests in the first place.

Let us then suppose that a person has an aunt which is discovered to have an incurable cancer. Let us moreover suppose that this aunt is in constant pain. In that case it would be unfair against this aunt, in the view of most people, to take her to a doctor, and ask him to give her a painless death. Those who did, would be accused of horrible things. Those who did not, would certainly not be accused of egoism and for not putting the aunt's best interests in the first place.

Why is this? The difference in attitudes that we have to human beings and to animals may be explained historically by referring to influence from stoicism and Christianity. We respect the dignity and integrity of human beings more than of animals. Concerning animals, we attach greater importance to minize suffering. But I am not sure that this difference can be justified in a rational way.

Such differences in attitudes are examples of facts which have to be taken into account in the ethical analysis. It is also possible that such attitudes can explain the importance which in different ethical codes has been attached to the requirement of informed consent, which will be discussed below.

Two methodological remarks

In ethical analysis several things are important. First, I want to stress the importance of methodology as a description of how to proceed step by step in order to identify, clarify, and solve problems. This is important since vested interests of various kinds can parade as ethical interests.

The best method to discover the problems is in my view to identify the main parties involved, describe their rational interests (defined in terms of what they would choose if informed about relevant facts and given a chance to think about the matter), and then locate potential and actual conflicts of interests.

There are a number of parties involved in epidemiological research: The research subjects (individuals as well as the population studied as a whole), present as well as future patients which may benefit from the research, the employers of the research subjects, the community in which they live, health agents (including policy makers as well as administrators) the researchers and their institutes, the scientific community at large, those funding the research, which may be research councils, communities and corporations (which may have rather different long range interests), mass media, trade unions and various interest groups, the general public (including tax payers).

We must not pretend that conflicts of interests never occur between these parties. In the literature there are several attempts to suggest how such conflicts should be handled, attempts which go beyond the scope of this paper.

The second important thing is the role of dialogue in ethical analysis. It is essential to create a possibility for the people concerned to exchange views in mutual respect. This has to do with the simple fact that ethics is a different kind of subject than mathematics, and we must take seriously the possibility that in a number of matters, people can have different norms and values.

Sometimes it turns out that differences in attitudes will disappear when the parties involved get the facts straight, sometimes they depend on misunderstandings. Sometimes desires and aversions can be changed by cognitive psychotherapy of the sort described by Richard Brandt. But this can only happen if they first are allowed to be tested against each other in an open and free dialogue where each voice has an equal chance. It then becomes important to specify the conditions for the ideal dialogue situation - a work which has been carried out energetically by the German philosopher Jurgen Habermas.

Informed consent in research

It is well known that the requirement of informed consent is vague and problematic in many ways. The distinction between informed and misinformed consent (respectively not-consent) is not always as clear in practice as it is on paper.

Nevertheless, it is easy to see that more and more importance has been attached to informed consent in ethical codes from the declaration of Helsinki to the declaration of Hawaii. But epidemiologists find this requirement troublesome, as do people in the social sciences carrying out longitudinal studies. This has to do with the special characteristics of epidemiological research which Peter Allebeck in his paper has discussed so well. When information in very large data files is to be used, "informed consent is not a realistic option", writes professor Last.

Perhaps a distinction between two senses in which one can participate in a study would help. By qualified (or active) participation I mean taking part in interviews, experiments, or answer questionnaires. Here informed consent is obviously justified. By non-qualified (or passive) participation I mean being the subject of study without knowing it, e.g. a study of information collected in data files. Here it is an open question whether information consent is ethically called for; this may depend on the nature of the data, the way they are stored, the methods used in the analysis, and the extent to which data of different types are combined.

There is a slight, but interesting, difference in the choice of words by professor Last and professor Allebeck. The latter writes that "epidemiological methods... are not really covered by the Helsinki declaration". But professor Last writes that "work with human subjects requires adherence to a code of ethical conduct, such as the Helsinki declaration" and that "Epidemiologists honour this declaration".

It is important to distinguish between what is practical or expedient and what is ethical. It is one thing to say that informed consent is impractical, and hence it is ethical not to require informed consent. And it is something quite different to say that to insist on informed consent in certain types of investigations can cause unnessecary embarrasment, make important research impossible, cause systematic nonresponse and thereby make the results of the research misleading. For example, this may be the case in certain kinds of criminological studies as well as in studies on HIV/Aids, on drug abuse, sexual perversions, violence in the family, or abuse of children.

If political decisions are based on such research, this may give rise to many bad decisions and hence violate the principle of non-maleficience. In that case we have an ethical argument against the requirement of informed consent. It is this latter line of thought which should be explored and illustrated by specific examples.

I think it should be possible to work towards a two-step solution. First, split up the requirement of informed consent into two: a requirement of information and a requirement of consent. Then specify the conditions under which one or both or neither of these requirements should be satisfied. Are the data sensitive? Are they stored in a way that endangers confidentiality? Can individuals be identified in the course of analysis? Are they combined with other sensitive data? If these questions are answered by no, it may be unnecessary to ask for consent. If information will only cause unnecessary embarrasment and lead to a systematic non-response in an important study, it may even be unnecessary to inform.

It is important that ethical committees or review boards decide in each particular case if, when, how, by whom, to whom, from whom information should be given and/or consent be obtained. Naturally, the research team has a vested interest here, and the experience in Sweden, particularly after the debate on the research project called Metropolit shows how important it is to keep the confidence of the general public, and what happens when this confidence is lost.

Sometimes it may be enough that the committee is informed, other times information could be given via mass media, sometimes each individual research subject should be informed. In still other cases, it may be possible to presume consent and give those who do not want to participate a chance to opt out. Sometimes consent should be given by each individual, at other times by proxies or representatives of the research subjects, sometimes not at all.

Feedback is important, and it is possible to present summaries of main findings in mass media or on information sheet which can be distributed to the population studied. Something rather like this has been tried with very good results in the Tierp project in Sweden.

What sort of people should be on ethical committees, what sort of competence and experience should they have, and how should the committees work? Such questions will then turn out to be important.

For example, it can hardly be reasonable to have people working as nurses or curators in the health care as laymen; they are not laymen in a strict sense. They should be on ethical committees, but not as laymen. At the same time it is important that the committees have a possibility to call in people, so that each controversial question can be discussed under the best possible conditions, and that no important information is withheld or missing.

Special problems in this regard are raised by so-called mixed studies, where interviews or examinations are combined with information collected from existing records. Since the meaning of what is said may take on a special significance in the light of these data, the researcher should always, in such cases, inform the research subject about his plans to follow up the interview by collecting other types of data, or tell the research subject that he already has such information.

The status of ethical standards

Who shall set the ethical standards? Perhaps one ought to pause a moment and ask whether it is at all the case that some should set ethical standards for others. Perhaps ethical standards rather should develop in a dialogue between the parties involved along the lines indicated earlier.

In this dialogue the parties should train their abilities to consider long-term consequences, to vary the scenario for the future, including empirical and normative assumptions, and to change position ("if I were you and you were me") in accordance with the ethics of reciprocity, which is such a conspicuous and important part in many cultures and ethical thoughts, from those of Confucius to those of Kant and Hare. This is not to say that all conflicts will automatically disappear, if this strategy is followed, but that it will be more easy to agree on what one disagrees about.

Should ethical standards be regarded as a matter of cultural customs or should they be universally applied? This is one of questions to be considered in this session. Personally, I believe (like John Mackie) that ethical guidelines have an instrumental value. We invent them in order to be able to better satisfy certain important human needs. This does not lessen the importance of these guidelines. What could be more important than to improve the possibilities of the human race to survive the various threats it imposes on itself?

Today we can witness two tendencies: on the one hand increased pluralism, increased cultural and national awareness, which is illustrated in so many ways in the third world and in the Soviet Union. On the other hand we face the increasing internationalism of science. Scientific cooperation across national borders increases, as does the number of multicenter studies. Data are exported and imported across national boundaries.

This internationalisation is not only due to improved communications but also to the fact that fatal diseases like cancer and AIDS seldom respect national boundaries but require cooperation between researchers from different countries. To make such cooperation possible, it becomes important to work along the lines suggested by both professor Last and professor Keyserlingk to establish ethical guidelines dealing with specific problems.

Responsibility of researchers and of politicians

It is sometimes necessary to strike a balance between competing interests. It is on the one hand clear that information about fatal diseases and serious risks must be passed on to those concerned. But on the other hand it is clear that one wants to avoid unnecessary worries about vaguely known possible risks, particularly in view of the hazards that a diagnostic test may involve, and the unnecessary anguish created by false positives. But who decides which worries, and whose worries, are unnecessary?

If the positions taken by politicians are not to be shortsighted and opportunistic, it is necessary that researchers become involved in an open information about what epidemiological research is, how it is carried out, and why it is important. By information I do not mean lobbying behind closed doors, but explanation of what epidemiology is about - including not only who benefits from epidemiological research, but also which, if any, the hazards are. This information has to be concrete and given in such a way that the general public, as well as politicians, can understand the issues. This includes information about what (and whose) interests are threatened, if such restrictions are imposed on this research that it cannot survive.

Politicians naturally want to be reelected, sometimes for unselfish reasons: they will not be able to carry on the work they have initiated for the public good. It is then tempting to become oversensitive to trends and pressure of opinion from mass media and various interest groups. Owing to such pressure, and the fear of a society of the sort described by Orwell in 1984, several important data files have been dismantled and cannot any longer be used for longitudinal studies, also in Sweden.

Possible conflicts between principles

Sometimes these conflicts between the principle of autonomy and other basic bio-ethical principles are erroneously represented as conflicts between the interests of society and those of the individual. In an age of increasing individualism, such a presentation is politically biased - against epidemiological research. In a fight between David and Goliath, our sympathies tend to be on the side of David.

Besides, who is society? It is ourselves and our children. There is rather a conflict between the interests of different groups and individuals, and sometimes between the short-term and long-term interests of the same individual or group.

In the short run I may be interested in being left alone. But I may realize that in a longer perspective it will be in my own rational interest to have information about environmental problems, and reliable statistics concerning the relation between pollution of water, air and the spread of e.g. cancer. It may also be in my own best interest that there is a well functioning planning of health care, and that the resources available are used in the best way possible - simply because I may need this in order to be able to live a good life.

Ethics and social philosophy

What makes these conflicts between basic ethical principles particularly difficult to handle is that there is no obvious ranking order between these principles. The thesis that they ought to be ranked in one way rather than another is itself an ethical principle. The question then becomes how that principle is to be justified. If the principles are ranked in one way, we get one kind of society; if they are ranked in another way, we get a different kind of society. For example, in a libertarian society, the principle of autonomy is at the top, in a egalitarian society, the top position is held by the principle of justice, and in an utilitarian society, the principle of beneficience is the top principle.

The issue is then transformed to a choice between different types of society, and in that case ethical conflicts are related to the social views of the parties involved, in the same way that they often are related to, and based on, their view on man. Here is an interesting connection between ethics and political philosophy. For these reasons, guidelines rather than strict formal codes of conduct may be a realistic option.

Is it possible to argue for or against ideals of sociey in a rational way? It is possible. But there is also the danger of being caught in question-begging arguments of the type: we argue for a collectivistic or utilitarian society, where the principle of beneficience is given priority over the principle of autonomy for the reason that this in the long run will increase the possibilities for human beings to live a good life. But what does this good life consist in? This should then settle the issue. Those who stand on different sides of the fence are, however, likely to have radically different ideas or visions about this.

Why guidelines or codes of conduct

There is an interesting difference between what I take to be the position of professor Last and that of professor Keyserlingk. Professor Last appears to be in favor of guidelines which "state the positions that could be adopted in certain situations" rather that a formal code of conduct.

This seems to be somewhat different from what professor Keyserlingk argues for. He wants both the more general and the more specific ethical guidelines to have normative validity; "to conclude otherwise", he writes, "would to be to betray the letter and the spirit of the many UN and WHO health related Codes and Constitutions, which are meant to be universally applied and provide no exceptions for particular cultures or societies."

Perhaps the difference between these two speakers should not be exaggerated. Personally I am more pessimistic than professor Keyserlingk about the possibility of getting people from different cultures to agree on specific guidelines with normative validity. The process that leads to acceptance of ethical guidelines will have a great educational value; and this process may turn out to be more important than the final written document.

Anyway, to say that a code with vague rules, or rules which state the positions which <u>could</u> be taken, without prescribing one of them, should be applied universally is not to say that a specific and precise rule should be universally applied.

<u>Concluding remarks</u>

Towards the end of his paper, professor Last mentions a number of reasons which have been used against guidelines or codes of conducts for epidemiologists. To support the thesis that the moral position of the epidemiologist would be strengthened by such a code, I would like to comment on some of the arguments.

For example, the second reason mentioned by professor Last is stated as follows: "epidemiologists belong to professional groups who adhere to an existing code". This, of course, is no objection if that code does not discuss the particular problems raised by epidemiological research methods.

The third reason mentioned by professor Last is that: "confusion would result from yet another code, especially if its clauses differed from those of existing codes." But here it is important to realize that "different" does not entail "incompatible"; it is only incompatible clauses that create genuine confusion.

A fourth reason mentioned by professor Last is stated as follows: "a code would be unenforcible". But suppose that no research money would be given to projects which have not been found by an ethics committee or a review board to be compatible with the guidelines of such a code. Suppose, moreover, that the results of such a research would not be published in prestigeous medical journals unless it had been first approved by such a committee. In that case it would be reasonable to say that the code could be "enforced" without misusing that word.

Here I would also like to call attention to some problems raised but not solved by professor Keyserlingk. His point about the need for educational assistance is obviously important, but there is nevertheless the problem of who draws the line between adaption and compromise of essentials ("allow as much adaption as possible short of compromising the essentials").

Like Peter Allebeck, I would like to conclude that only if a good ethical conduct is maintained in epidemiological studies will it be possible to prevent that restrictions of administrative and legal nature are imposed on such studies. But again, there is a difference between saying that epidemiologists should be ethical to avoid restrictions, and saying that they should maintain a certain conduct because otherwise they would violate certain widely accepted ethical principles in our culture.

References

1. Beauchamp, T., and Childress, J.: Principles of biomedical ethics, Second ed. New York and Oxford: Oxford University Press, 1983.

2. Brandt, R.: A theory of the good and the right. Oxford: Clarendon, 1979.

3. Habermas, J.: Vorbereitende bemerkungen zu einer theorie der kommunikativen kompetenz, in Habermas and Luhman, eds, Theorie der gesellschaft oder sozial-technologie. Frankfurt am Main: Suhrkamp, 1971.

4. Hare, R.M.: Moral thinking. Oxford: Clarendon, 1981.

5. Hermerén, G.: Kunskapens pris. Stockholm: Humanistisk samhällsvetenskapliga forskningsrådet, 1986.

6. Kant, I.: Grundlegung zur metaphysik der Sitten. Hamburg: Meiner, (1785) 1957.

7. Mackie, J.: Ethics, inventing right and wrong. London and Harmondsworth: Penguin, (1977) 1987.

8. Gillon, R.: Philosophical medical ethics. New York: Wiley, 1985.

Ethics in Medicine, edited by
Peter Allebeck and Bengt Jansson.
Raven Press, New York © 1990.

ETHICAL ASPECTS ON HIV

INTRODUCTION

Bengt Jansson

As HIV infection actualizes most ethical issues met with in medicine it is natural to devote a special section of this book to ethical aspects on HIV.

Dr Mary Jeanne Kreek, working with research on drug abuse in New York, stresses in her paper the paramount importance of prevention, intervention and treatment as well as research related to parenteral drug abuse and AIDS. Failure to address all aspects of this combined medical problem should be considered to be unethical. For instance, methadone maintenance programs have shown themselves to be efficient in reducing the number of addicts seropositive for HIV antibody. A problem, however, which is not easily solved, is the maintenance of confidentiality in handling HIV patients.

Dr Barbro Westerholm will give a background to the differences in approach to HIV from the medical profession and from the politicians. The reaction from the politicians is similar to a crisis reaction and has now reached the fourth stage, the phase of reorientation. Dr Westerholm also discusses the ethical issues of exchange of needles and syringes. Her attitude towards such exchange programs is positive and she agrees with a statement from the Swedish Medical Association that it is up to the physician to decide what is best for the patients.

Dr Ove Berglund approaches the issue in a very practical way, describing eight short case histories, each of them presenting different ethical problems. According to dr Berglund compulsory testing of large populations or groups does not necessarily lead to diminished spread of the virus. A primary goal for the doctor, in his or her relation to the patient, is to protect the patient's integrity. There may arise situations where it is better to disregard the law than to lose the patient's confidence.

Dr Tore Nilstun will present a model designed to identify and analyse ethical conflicts. He discusses the four ethical principles autonomy, non-maleficence, beneficence and justice. Sometimes the understanding goes far enough as to solve the conflicts. But in most cases, and that is the main value of the model, the understanding helps to overcome the paralyzing feeling of facing an unresolvable dilemma.

Ethics in Medicine, edited by
Peter Allebeck and Bengt Jansson.
Raven Press, New York © 1990.

HIV INFECTION AND PARENTERAL DRUG ABUSE: ETHICAL ISSUES IN DIAGNOSIS, TREATMENT, RESEARCH AND THE MAINTENANCE OF CONFIDENTIALITY

Mary Jeanne Kreek

Since 1986, the World Health Organization has officially recognized the world-wide spread of HIV infections and AIDS disease, which has reached epidemic proportions in many regions, and also has recognized the magnitude of the relationship of HIV infection and AIDS disease to parenteral drug abuse, as well as to other risk factors. The numerous and diverse ethical issues raised by HIV infection and especially by its prevalence in parenteral drug abusers are increasingly recognized, discussed, and addressed in public policy decisions and yet often remain unresolved.

Figure 1. HIV infection and parenteral drug abuse: Ethical issues

Diagnosis
Treatment
Research
Maintenance of confidentiality

The disease entity of AIDS was first identified

and clinically described in 1981. In retrospect, HIV infection entered the parenteral drug abusing population of heroin addicts in New York City around 1975, with a rapid increase in prevalence in seropositivity for the HIV antibody, and thus the emergence of an epidemic, from 1978 to 1984. In studies of both active intravenous heroin addicts and also former heroin addicts in methadone maintenance treatment performed by our group and also by the group of Des Jarlais at the New York State Division of Substance Abuse Services in1984 to 1985, a time when specific serologic tests for HIV antibody were being developed and validated, we found and reported that whereas 50 to 60% of street heroin addicts were seropositive for HIV antibody, less than 10% of patients who had entered effective methadone maintenance treatment programs prior to the AIDS epidemic reaching New York in 1978 were seropositive for the HIV antibody.

These findings immediately raised ethical issues concerning the clinical needs for expanded effective treatment resources for heroin addiction, as well as other types of parenteral drug abuse, ideally programs combining both pharmacological (or nonpharmacological) treatment for the primary drug addiction problem i.e., heroin addiction, as well as nonpharmacological treatment for other drug abuse problems, and other medical and behavioral treatment services, along with appropriate counseling, rehabilitation efforts, and AIDS risk reduction education. Research studies of this type also raised ethical issues with respect to individual diagnosis of HIV infection, and the determination of the prevalence of HIV infection within a defined group of unidentified individuals, in both clinical and more basic research settings.

Figure 2. Diagnosis by anti-HIV-1 testing.

A. Impact on patient

    1. Positive

    A) Knowledge of whether or not infected; removal of uncertainty.

    B) Possible early entry into treatment, if positive.

2. Negative

A) Psychological/emotional impact negative, if test is positive, in an addicted patient, at best, in the process of recovering from drug addiction, and at worst, not yet in treatment.

B) Potential breech of confidentiality with resultant "double jeopardy", ie. drug abuse and HIV infection.

B.   Impact on society

1. Identification of infected persons and possible reduced risk of spread of infection.

The greatest risk group for AIDS disease and also HIV infection is the group defined as intravenous drug abusers or parenteral drug abusers, in New York City, New Jersey, as well as several locations in Europe. This risk group of parenteral drug abusers is also the most rapidly growing risk group, with the numbers of new cases of AIDS in the current overall first risk group, homosexual males, now plateauing or declining. Therefore prevention, intervention, treatment, as well as research related to parenteral drug abuse and AIDS is of paramount importance. Failure to address all aspects of this combined medical problem should be considered to be unethical.

Figure 3. Treatment of drug abuse: treatment of HIV infection or AIDS.

A.   Impact on patient

1) Treatment of drug addiction may break cycle of abuse, reduce criminality and allow restoration of normal lifestyle.
Treatment may allow normalization of physiological processes disrupted by drug addiction. Successful treatment seems more probable if specific pharmacological treatment is avail able.

2) Treatment of early symptomatic or silent HIV infection (with T4 helper cell absolute count < 500 cells) with AZT may prolong symptom free interval and slow rate of progression to AIDS treatment of AIDS may prolong life.

B. Impact on society

1) Treatment of drug abuse may decrease spread of HIV infection, especially the heterosexual spread and spread to babies. Treatment may also reduce criminality.

2) Treatment of drug abuse and of HIV infection will initially make great demands on society, especially in the identification of sites for treatment and also by demanding large numbers of skilled and diverse staff.

3) Treatment will be expensive, but should be cost effective in 5 to 10 years.

At this time there are increasing numbers of therapeutic agents which may retard the progression of HIV infection to AIDS or may reduce or treat various medical complications which define or complicate HIV infection or AIDS disease. These different therapeutic agents may or may not result in an overall improvement of the quality of life. However, with the increasing availability of these agents, the ethical issues concerning the identification and especially early identification, of HIV infection must be raised again.

Figure 4. Research related to HIV infection and parenteral drug abuse: Ethical issues.

Further research efforts on available, as well as on potential new therapeutic agents, and also other types of basic laboratory, basic clinical and applied clinical research related to HIV infection and AIDS disease are sometimes confounded by well-intended policies to address ethical issues, including the major issue of confidentiality, as related to such studies. These ethical and confidentiality issues are further complicated in studies of combined HIV infection and addictive diseases.

Treatment needs for both drug addiction and also AIDS disease, for those persons who are intravenous drug addicts in the United States, primarily heroin addicts, and who also have HIV infection or have AIDS disease, are raising many complicated ethical issues. Issues related to "responsibility" including "responsibility" for acquisition of each of these diseases, and responsibility for prevention of further spread of these diseases by the individual afflicted, and in counter-balance, "responsibility" of society for prevention of these diseases and responsibility for their treatment have yet to be resolved.

Parenteral drug abusers are the primary sources for spread of HIV infection to the heterosexual population and also to children prior to or at birth. At this time, the magnitude of the HIV infection problem in all possible various groups of persons who might be exposed remains unknown, primarily because of various ethical issues. Possibly the greates ethical issues complicating all aspects of diagnosis, treatment and research, in the parenteral drug abuser (in the past as well at the present time) and in the HIV infected person or patient with AIDS disease, and especially when these two disorders occur concomitantly, are issues related to confidentiality.

Figure 5. Maintenance of confidentility.

A. Appropriate maintenance of confidentiality is the major ethical issue with respect to HIV infection and drug addiction at this time.

B. Fear of breach of confidentiality is important with respect to

1) Diagnosis of HIV infection and drug abuse.

2) Treatment of HIV infection and drug abuse.

3) Related research needs.

C. Confidentiality is now breached routinely accidentally in the process of federal and third party reimbursement and peer review of health care, and in the process of conducting public health measures to reduce spread of HIV infection.

Public policy and legal guidelines to protect confidentiality have often unintentionally impeded diagnosis, treatment and research efforts in these areas.

Many of these confidentiality issues are not unique to parenteral drug abuse and HIV infection, but are issues of greater individual and public concern in this setting. Resolution of these confidentiality issues would undoubtedly facilitate basic and clinical research, diagnosis, treatment and prevention efforts and would thus benefit both the individual afflicted with parenteral drug abuse and HIV infection and would also benefit society as a whole.

References

1. Des Jarlais, D.C., Marmor, M., Cohen, H. et al: Antibodies to a retrovirus etiologically associated with Acquired Immunodeficiency Syndrome (AIDS) in populations with increased incidences of the syndrome. Morbidity and Mortality Weekly Report, 33:377-379, 1984.

2. Novick, D., Kreek, M.J., Des Jarlais, D. et al: Antibodyto LAV, the putative agent of AIDS, in parenteral drug abusers and methadone-maintained patients: Abstract of clinical research findings: Therapeutic, historical, and ethical aspects.
In: Problems of Drug Dependence, 1985: Proceedings of the 47th Annual Scientific Meeting of The Committee on Problems of Drug Dependence. Harris, L.S., ed., NIDA Research Monograph Series., Rockville, MD., DHHS Publication No. (ADM)86-1448 67:318-320, 1986.

3. Des Jarlais, D.C., Friedman, S.R., Novick, D.M. et al: HIV I Infection among intravenous drug users in Manhattan, New York City 1977 to 1987. J Am Med Ass 261:1008-1012, 1989.

4. Dole, V.P., Nyswander, M.E. and Kreek, M.J.: Narcotic blockade. Arch Intern Med., 118:304-309, 1966.

5. Kreek, M.J.: Medical safety and side effects of methadone in tolerant individuals. J Amer Med Ass, 223:665-668, 1973.

6. Kreek, M.J.: Multiple drug abuse patterns and medical consequences. In: Psychopharmacology: The Third Generation of Progress. Meltzer, H.Y., ed. 1597-1604, 1987.

7. Novick, D.M., Khan, I., Kreek, M.J.: Acquired immunodeficiency syndrome and infection with hepatitis viruses in individuals abusing drugs by injfection. United Nations Bulletin on Narcotics 1986;38:15-25.

8. Novick, D.M., Ochshorn, M., Ghali, V., Croxson,

T.S., Mercer, W.D., Chiorazzi, N., Kreek, M.J.: Natural killer cell activity and lymphocyte subsets in parenteral heroin abusers and long-term methadone maintenance patients. J Pharm Exper Ther 1989;250: 606-620.

Ethics in Medicine, edited by
Peter Allebeck and Bengt Jansson.
Raven Press, New York © 1990.

MEDICAL VERSUS POLITICAL ASPECTS OF CREATING A POLICY AGAINST A SEVERE DISASTER

Barbro Westerholm

As physician, scientist, former administrator, politician and chairperson of a non-governmental organization I have been involved in policymaking. I have among other things been part of a system creating a policy against a severe disaster, that is the HIV-epidemic.

I have witnessed how conflicts have arisen between different groups of people. I have witnessed how these conflicts have delayed and hampered decision-making necessary in order to combat the epidemic. Resources have been wasted and political and medical goals have been opposing each other.

I have tried to understand why all this has taken place. I want to believe that all involved wanted to do their best for the society and its individuals.

In this paper I make an attempt to elucidate some of the factors behind these phenomena and I will make some suggestions how to get around the difficulties.

As a first step I think it is important to analyze

the conditions precedent for the medical profession on one side and the politicians on the other.

Conditions precedent for the medical profession

From time immemorial the medical profession has aimed at giving the patients the treatment which according to scientific evidence and medical experience has proven to be the most effective and least dangerous. Mistakes have led to punishment.

The oldest ethical rules for medical action are found in the Oath of Hippocrates (460 B C). The two basic paragraphs read:

"The regiment I adopt shall be for the benefit of my patients according to my ability and judgement, and nor for their hurt or for any wrong. I will give no deadly drug to any, though it be asked me, nor will I counsel such.

Whatsoever house I enter, there will I go for the benefit of the sick, refraining from all wrongdoing or corruption, and especially from any act of seduction, of male or female, of bond or free. Whatsoever things I see or hear concerning the life of men, in my attendance on the sick or even apart therefrom, which ought not to be noised abroad, I will keep silence thereon, counting such things to be as sacred secrets".

Since then different oaths, principles and guidelines have been developed by the medical profession in various parts of the world.

The first international rules were presented as late as 1948 following the horrifying experiences from the Second World War. That was the year when the Declaration of Geneva was developed. It was accepted by the World Health Organization the following year. The basic paragraphs read:

- "The health of my patients will be my first consideration".

- "I will not permit considerations of religion, nationality, race, party politics or social standing to intervene between my duty and my patient".

The Declaration of Geneva has thereafter been followed by other declarations giving ethical norms for psychiatrists, for clinical research, testing of medicines, doctors relation to torture and other inhuman acts etc.

Thus, the activity of the physicians should be based on medical science, medical experience and the ethical norms which have been established as support and protection of the patients. The role of the physician is to treat, palliate, console and prevent disease. "Primum est non nocere" - the primary goal is not to harm - is the leading principle since ancient times.

Conditions precedent for the politicians

The politician's responsibility is to institute laws, develop strategies and policies, impose taxes and distribute tax money according to policies and priorities agreed on. The application of the legislation falls upon the administrators and other professional groups involved.

The borderline between the politicians and the professionals appears clear but occasionally conflicts of interest appear. This can be exemplified by the "HIV/Aids story" in Sweden.

The medical profession and HIV

When the first Swedish cases of Aids were reported to the National Board of Health and Welfare the cause of the disease was not known. The governmental agency closely followed the development but was entirely dependent on the information it obtained via scientific and medical channels. The extensiveness of the problem was suspected but it was not until physicians meeting the patients described the reality to the decision makers that action was taken to fight the severe disaster, the spread of HIV. An extra push was given by scientists involved in viral and closely related research and by representatives of the risk groups. A good communication between administrative decision makers, the medical profession and representatives of the risk groups was vital for the establishment of a policy against HIV.

Of importance in the policy making was later the association Physicians against Aids which was established in 1984 by a small group of physicians with experience in epidemiology, infectious diseases, venereology and gynecology, drug abuse and homosexual behaviour. It was obvious, early on, that it was important to claim the HIV-infection as a medical matter and not allow it to become a political issue as this could hamper a direct approach to the difficult questions arisen by the infection. In order to bring about such a development it was felt that this could only be possible by the establishment of an association of physicians covering all the different medical fields involved to achieve general acceptance. These physicians acted and still act besides their ordinary work as a pressure group targeting at their colleagues, patients, politicians and other decisions makers. They were among the first to spread facts about the disease to other health care personnel, the public, homosexuals and addicts. Since the HIV-infection in Sweden first struck homosexual men it proved necessary and important to increase the knowledge about and the understanding of homosexuality among health care personnel.

The association has as a main goal to minimize the spread of the HIV-infection, to increase resources for clinical research with new drugs and to minimize the suffering and damage caused by HIV both to individual patients and to the society as a whole. The unique tools are knowledge and experience and above all compassion.

The politicians and HIV

The reaction of the politicians and administrative decision-makers when HIV was first described bears resemblance with the reaction seen in patients when they first learn to know that they suffer from a deadly disease e.g. cancer.

In the initial moment they saw the width of the problem which quickly led them into a shock phase. The second phase with denial and diminishment of the problem followed: "It cannot be true. Nothing such can happen to us now when we can cure so much". When the risk groups had been identified: homosexuals, addicts and haemophiliacs a kind of relief was expressed: "It is them, not us who are hit".

Gradually politicians and administrators came into the third phase when they saw the reality and listened attentively to knowledge and advice presented to them by the medical world but much time had been lost at the beginning. The demand for action was heavy both from the public, the physicians and the risk groups and their associations. There was no limitation of how much money could be spent on information campaigns. A special committee was established headed by the Minister of Health and Social Welfare composed by politicians from different parties and experts. The task was wide: besides information campaigns legislative but also pure medical matters were dealt with.

We are now in the fourth phase: the phase of reorientation. HIV/Aids is no longer on the headlines. One has got used to the fact that we get one new case per day. The worst prognoses have not become true, much because of the preventive work which has been performed. Danger is felt to be over. Other matters like taxation, nuclear power and the fate of the environment attract more interest.

But this calm period was preceeded by a turbulent time when the strategies and policies to combat HIV collided with the policies against drug abuse.

HIV and drug abuse

There is no disagreement between the medical profession and the politicians that the goal of the work against drug abuse is to create a society free of narcotics. Strong action is needed to accomplish this. The drug addicts have to be supported in their endeavours to cease abusing narcotic drugs.

In this work the health care personnel plays an important role. At the same time it is also responsible for the prevention of the spread of infections diseases including HIV in society, among drug addicts. And drug addicts have the same right to good health care as other people in Sweden.

Exchange of needles and syringes

Certain diseases like hepatitis and HIV are to a great extent spread among addicts via the sharing of dirty needles and syringes. It is one of the most important ways by which HIV is spread.

It is against this background that needle and syringe exchange programmes have been established in many parts of the world in order to diminish the use of dirty tools and prevent the spread of HIV via intravenous injections.

In many countries it is possible to buy syringes and needles without restrictions in pharmacies while in Sweden a prescription is needed to obtain them.

The World Health Organization has recommended the member states to make clean needles and syringes available for the addicts. In Sweden the Swedish Medical Association, the Swedish Society of Medicine, the Association of Psychiatrists, Physicians against Aids, the Medical Ethical Committee of the Government as well as some patient organizations are in favour of such an exchange programme. The experience from a needle exchange project in southern Sweden (1) has given positive experience. Besides clean tools the addicts also obtain information how to protect themselves against HIV. The spread of HIV among them has been almost negligable while in Stockholm more than half of the intravenous addicts are now HIV-positive. Another positive effect of the project was that it attracted drug addicts who were previously unknown some of which later asked for help to treat their addiction.

The matter of access to clean needles and syringes was brought up in Parliament. The majority of politicians in Parliament voted for such far-going restrictions of future needle and syringe exchange programmes that they will not be meaningful to conduct. Stockholm for instance where most of the addicts live, should not be included in the programme. According to the decision taken by Parliament it is not possible for a physician to hand out a clean syringe and needle to an intravenous drug abuser in order to prevent the spread of HIV despite convincing medical evidence that such a mesure can contribute to the prevention of the spread of HIV.

This creates a dilemma for the medical profession. Should it follow the medical principles set out by WHO and other medical - professional organizations or should it obey the politicians. A clear answer has been presented by the Swedish Medical Association: "The physician's work must be ruled by a humanitarian attitude towards Man. They are guided by the ethical principles of the Association which in a turn are based on the internationally accepted rules and principles. These means that it is up to the physician to decide what is best for the patient."

I wholeheartedly agree with this attitude. What is going to happen now? Most likely a physician will break the political decision and report himself to the Board of Malpractice in order to get the matter settled legally.

Methadone

The other conflicting issue is methadone treatment of drug addicts who have failed to stop drug abuse despite several attempts.

The approved indications for use of methadone in Sweden is severe pain, e.g. cancer pain. If methadone is to be used to treat addicts the addict has to be accepted in a methadone programme. Very strict inclusion criteria have been developed and there is a political decision on how many patients in Sweden who can be included in the methadone programme. This number does not correspond to the needs. At present there sig a waiting list up to two years depending on in which area of Sweden the addict lives. During this time there is a great risk that the addict both contracts HIV and spread it further.

To the medical profession this is an inacceptable situation particularly since the suicide rate is also increased in the group of addicts waiting for methadone (2).

Priority conflicts

It is obvious that the politicians here were only able to deal with one policy at a time. When there was a conflict they ranked drug abuse first since the problem in numbers at present is greater than HIV-infection. They disregard from the fact that HIV is an incurable, deadly disease spread by a virus via blood and sexual intercourse. History has taught us that sexually transmitted diseases are the most difficult to prevent. Drug abuse on the other hand is a severe health problem but it can be cured although it is difficult.

The way forward

The first obligation of the medical profession is to provide a good care for the patients. In order to reach this goal the physician has to use his knowledge and experience and constantly update himself with regard to new findings. He also has a responsibility to alert the politicians and other decisions makers about the disaster and communicate his knowlegde and advice how to handle the situation. He has to suggest strategies to prevent the disaster from spread and how to best care for the already infected.

The politicians on their side have a responsibility to listen and act on the basis of what they learn. They should base their strategies on the reality and not on ideological theoretical beliefs. Their task is to find ways and means to prevent the disaster to spread in society and to make resources available to care for the ones who have been hit. They have also an important role to play when forming attitudes towards a health risk. A premature statement on trends and risks can ruin a well-planned health promotion activity.

Physicians on the other hand should respect the situation of the politicians who are usually involved in a number of very different questions and decisions which sometimes are in conflict with each other. The physicians should be aware of the fact that politicians usually are healthy workoholics with little or no experience of working with and for people in crisis.

To listen, to communicate, to build up respect fo each other's experience and situation is fundamental for both physicians, scientists and politicians if we are to succeed in our efforts to create a healthy society.

Since politicians often listen more to members of their own group than experts outside some physicians might consider entering the political world. I think medical knowledge and experience of patient contacts and scientific work is badly needed among decision makers like politicians.

Concluding remark

In summary: in order to form a policy against a severe disaster, a good communication, respect for each other's, knowledge, experience and working conditions has to be established between the medical profession and politicians. Both have to follow the spirit of the Geneva declaration:

"The health and well-being of the people is my first consideration."

Furthermore I think politicians responsible for health care need to be exposed to medical ethics.

Many professional groups have developed ethical guidelines for their work. Besides the physicians engineers, psychologists, social workers and journalists have ethical professional codexes. I think it is high time to develope an ethical codex or ethical guidelines also for politicians. I have made an attempt and presented them elsewhere (3). Maybe these guidelines could be the subject for discussion at the next conference held by this group in two years time from now.

References

1. Ljungberg, B., Tunving, K., Andersson, B.: Rena sprutor till narkomaner. Studentlitteratur 1989. Lund, Sweden.

2. Grönbladh, L., Gunne, L.: Methadone assisted rehabilitation of Swedish heroin addicts. Drug and Alcohol Dependence. 1989;24:31-37.

3. Westerholm, B.: Etik i politiken. Liberal Debatt 1989;38-40.

ETHICAL ISSUES IN CLINICAL PRACTICE

Ove Berglund

The following are examples of ethical problems you meet as HIV/AIDS patient' doctor.

1. Your patient, a married man with two teen-aged sons, has not told his wife that he is HIV infected. One reason is that he does not dare to reveal that he has had a secret homosexual life with several anonymous contacts since 15 years. He has had sex with his wife infrequently, until he found out he was HIV infected. What actions, if any, will you take to inform his wife?

2. A sexual partner to a HIV positive person is offered a HIV test but refuses to take the test because he does not want to know the result. What shall I do? (A Swedish problem).

3. A young homosexual immigrant dies from AIDS and Kaposi sarcoma. He has told his parents, who are mormons, that he is seriously ill from cancer. Before he died he asked you several times not to disclose the AIDS diagnosis to his parents.

What will you write on the death certificate? What

will you tell his mother whom you meet for the first time a week after her son's death? What is your answer when the mother asks if he had AIDS?

4. A 72-year old man, who has gone through heart-surgery in the beginning of the 80s, has been traced as recipient of supposedly HIV infected blood. Should he be informed of the suspicion and offered a HIV test?

You happen to know that he has a good sexual relation with his 70 year old wife. Does this change the situation? Is the situation different if the couple is 40 years younger?

5. A nurse has during blood sampling accidentally injected some blood from an intravenous drug user into her own hand. If the patient is HIV positive she intends to take AZT for 6 weeks. The patient refuses to be tested.

6. An HIV positive person has not told his dentist about his condition because, if he does, he will most certainly be denied treatment. He argues (correctly) that several investigations show that dentists do not aquire HIV at their working chair. Should I support his arguing?

7. A surgeon refuses to operate a HIV infected patient because he is afraid to get contaminated. Is his refusal ethically acceptable? At what risk level can he refuse?

8. I offer my patient to join a 2-year placebo controlled study of a promising anti-HIV drug. The patient says that he might be dead in 2 years, he will absolutely not take placebo, he expects me to give him the promising drug, and he can accept any side effects, except death.

General discussion

It is reasonable to believe that a person who knows he is HIV infected is less likely to spread the virus than one who does not know. However, in my opinion a compulsory HIV testing is still unethical in almost every situation. Everyone has the right _not_ to know that he carries a deadly virus. When society enforces testing of any person it should be sure that this action prevents spread to another person or it should present arguments of similar strength.

Compulsory testing of large populations or groups do not necessarily lead to diminished spread of the virus. A "green card" system, which probably follows any compulsory testing program, gives a false and dangerous feeling of safety which in fact might be counter-productive.

I am convinced that HIV will establish itself in every society to a degree ("steady state") that is determined by the social and sexual patterns, the economic and hygienic standards, the drug culture etc of that society. Specific actions to prevent spread can be important in certain groups for short times but is no final solution as this requires more profound and stable cultural changes.

In my relation to the patient as a doctor a primary goal is to protect his integrity. In ethical conflicts between the society's and the patient's interests, which are quite uncommon, there may be situations where I disregard the law rather than to lose the patient's confidence. However, most ethical conflicts appear in the relation between the patient and his social environment, i.e. relatives, colleagues, medical personnel etc, and not between the patient and society's demands.

The ethical problems of research, e.g. drug trials, can be solved. When a potentially active drug with side effects is to be tried, the patient, unless very seriously ill, can accept placebo treatment for a limited time. After that time he is offered the active drug even before it has been proven active. A problem is the long study time, usually 2 years, before results are available.

To treat symptom free and non immunodeficient HIV infected persons with a potentially dangerous drug is problematic. However, studies of the natural history of HIV disease indicate that almost every infected person eventually becomes seriously ill. This means that most patients will accept considerable side effects.

Ethics in Medicine, edited by
Peter Allebeck and Bengt Jansson.
Raven Press, New York © 1990.

PUBLIC HEALTH MEASURES WITH HIV INFECTION: A MODEL FOR IDENTIFICATION AND ANALYSIS OF ETHICAL CONFLICTS

Tore Nilstun

The traditional methods used to check the spread of infectious diseases include surveillance for epidemiological purposes, screening of high-risk persons possibly exposed to infection, and isolation or quarantine of infected individuals. When used for attempting to control HIV infection these methods frequently give rise to ethical conflicts.

The purpose of this essay is to present and discuss a simple model helpful to identify and analyze such a conflicts. As an example I will use the ethical conflict described and analyzed by Lechaim Naggan in his contribution to the Second International Congress on Ethics in Medicine (1).

HIV screening tests

According to Naggan, all reports of official committees, whether from the Public Health Service, the Institute of Medicine or the Rand Corporation, advocate:

> Massive screening efforts in order to identify persons who are infected with HIV and to prevent transmission to the noninfected. Ideally, we should screen the whole population to be able to identify all those who are infected and to relieve the stigma of screening only high risk groups, who are already discriminated against (...). Epidemiologically, this does not make sense -high risk groups should be screened first. This is more cost-effective and is more likely to succeed than when one dilutes the effort on the low risk groups.

The purpose of screening tests for antibody to HIV is to identify infected individuals; to trace their sexual contacts and test them; offer them consultation on transmission to their sero-negative contacts. In consequence screening for HIV antibodies is a complex issue with implications that go beyond epidemiological reasoning.

Two of the ethical issues raised are described by Naggan:

> 1. In practically all screening programs, one has the ambition to offer the individual who is being screened some benefit. No such benefit (prevention or delay of onset of the disease) is available today for the HIV+. Hence there is no direct personal incentive to be screened.

> 2. On the contrary, our society is offering a disincentive for screening by its overt discrimination against AIDS patients and HIV+ individuals. Legislation in most states still considers most members of the high-risk groups as criminals. Job and school dicrimination is expected to be part of the risk one takes when one is being screened.

<u>Ethical conflicts</u>

An ethical conflict is a situation where there is, at the same time, a moral obligation for an agent to adopt each of two alternatives, the agent cannot adopt both alternatives together, and the agent can adopt each alternative separately (2).

In the situation described above there is,

according to Naggan, a moral obligation for health care professionals to do what is necessary to prevent transmission of HIV to those who are not infected. Massive screening is considered essential to achieve this end. But in the same situation there is also a moral obligation to respect the right to self-determination of those involved, which implies that only those who voluntarily accept screening should be tested. Each of the two alternatives are feasible. It is possible to do massive screening and it is possibleto respect autonomy. But in the present situation it is not possible to do both. Fear of discriminatory or legal actions are strong disincentives against voluntary testing - so strong that massive screening and respect for autonomy are not compatible.

A simple model

To facilitate the identification and analysis of such ethical conflicts I will introduce a simple model (Fig. 1). It combines ideas from Hermerén (3) and Francoeur (4). The model consists of two dimensions. The first dimension specifies the persons involved in the conflict to be analyzed. The second dimension specifies the relevant ethical principles, i.e. those principles which give rise to the moral obligations and moral rights of the persons involved.

Persons involved	Ethical principles			
	A	B	C	D
1				
2				
3				
4				

Figure 1. A model for identification and analysis of ethical conflicts.

In order to show the utility of this model I shall apply it to the situation described as an ethical conflict by Naggan.

The persons involved

The first task is to identify the persons involved in the situation. According to Naggan the total population is affected, but in particular he mentions the following: 1) health professionals (doctors, health educators, public health officials); 2) people who are HIV positive or have AIDS and their families and friends; 3) high-risk groups (homosexual men, intravenous drug users, prostitutes); and 4) ethnic minorities.

Not mentioned by Naggan, but probably presupposed, are sexual partners of those in high-risk groups; heterosexuals who have multiple partners; and young people emerging into the sphere of sexual activity and becoming potential customers in the illicit drug trade. In Naggan's description of the situation health care professionals are seen as agents who have conflicting obligations. It is from their perspective the conflict is viewed. All other persons are seen as affected.

Four ethical principles

The second task is to identify and formulate the relevant ethical principles. In my opinion, the choice should generally be determined by considering the values of all those involved in the conflict. The principles of autonomy, non-maleficence, beneficence and justice are widely recognized not only among moral philosophers and medical professionals, but also among the general public (5, 6). These principles, here quoted with minor modifications from The Appleton Consensus (7), will be used in my analysis:

Autonomy. All persons have a moral obligation to respect each other's autonomy insofar as such respect is compatible with the autonomy of all affected. The principle requires respect for the deliberated choices of those involved, their dignity and integrity.

Non-maleficence. All persons have a moral obligation not to harm each other. The infliction or risking of harm to others, can only be justified by the pursuit of some other moral value - principally benefits to those involved sufficient to outweigh the harm.

Beneficence. All persons have some moral obligation to benefit others, to some degree, especially those in need. Health care professionals have a particular obligation to benefit the public and to prevent harm.

Justice. All persons have a moral obligation to act justly or fairly to others. Health care professionals have a particular obligation to do so in the context of the distribution of social benefits and burdens, and in the context of respecting the rights of the public.

Naggan does not explicitly state the ethical principles used in his discussion. A possible explanation is that he, like many other medical professionals, is inclined towards situation ethics, i.e. the view that principles are of small value when ethical conflicts are to be solved because of the uniqueness of every situation (8). But it seems reasonable to ascribe to him something like the principles of autonomy, non-maleficence and beneficence. These three principles are all presupposed in his reasoning. No arguments are advanced that indicate that he would consider the principle of justice important in his analysis of mandatory screening.

Analysis

The third task is to place the persons involved in different groups. Each group should consist of persons who, in that particular situation, have similar moral obligations to fulfill or moral rights to be respected. The groups should be exhaustive, i.e. all persons involved should belong to at least one group. But the groups are not necessarily exclusive, i.e. one person may belong to more than one group.

For the present analysis four groups are needed. The first group, those who have to face the conflict, consists of the health care professionals. According to Naggan they have a moral obligation to respect the autonomy of the persons involved, not to harm them, and to prevent the spread of the epidemic.

The persons considered important to screen may be

divided into two subgroups: those who volunteer and those who do not volunteer. These two subgroups constitute the second and the third group respectively. According to Naggan mandatory screening violates the right to autonomy of those who do not volunteer. Both subgroups have, according to Naggan, a right not to be harmed as a result of testing.

All other persons being affected by the epidemic, i.e. the general public, constitute the fourth group. It is in the interest of the public that efficient measures are taken to prevent harm by stopping the spread of the epidemic. According to Naggan the public has a right to beneficence.

The fourth task is to sum up these moral obligations and moral rights in the model. Naggan, in his formulation of the conflict, emphasizes the moral obligation of health care professionals to respect the autonomy of those who do not consent to be tested, not to harm those who are tested (voluntarily or not), and by mandatory screening to prevent the harms of the epidemic.

To these rights and obligations I have added the right to **autonomy** of those who do consent (which might be violated in connection with or as a result of testing); the obligation of those worth screening to be tested, i.e. to be **beneficent**; the right to **justice** of those who do consent to be tested (they might feel that they carry an **unjust** burden of the prevention efforts), of those who do not consent (they should not be discriminated against), and of the general public (they have a right to be treated justly). (Fig. 2).

<u>A compromise</u>

The model is not designed to suggest any particular compromise. Further premises are needed in order to perform the fifth, and last step in the analysis, i.e. to solve the conflict. These premises are not only concerned with values, i.e. ethical

Groups of persons involved	Ethical principles			
	Autonomy	Non-maleficence	Beneficence	Justice
Health care professionals; doctors, nurses, etc	O	O	O	[O]
Persons worth testing who do consent	[R]	R	R [O]	[R]
Persons worth testing who do not consent	R	R	R [O]	[R]
Other people being affected by the epidemic			R	[R]

Figure 2. Analysis of the ethical conflict involved in mandatory screening for HIV in terms of moral obligations and moral rights. The letter "O" indicates that the principle gives rise to a relevant obligation, while the letter "R" indicates that the principle gives rise to a relevant right. Letters between brackets indicate that the obligations and rights are not mentioned by Naggan.

principles and their order of precedence, but also with facts about the situation, the conflicting alternatives and their consequences. I believe that knowledge of such facts is essential to rational discussions of ethical conflicts.

But rationality has its limits. In my opinion ethical principles are neither true nor false - "we are ourselves the ultimate and irrefutable arbiters of values" (9). The subjective biases of all ethical issues imply that there are no objectively correct solutions to ethical conflicts, only answers that satisfy the emotional and intellectual demands of particular individuals or groups.

The compromise suggested by Naggan is as follows:

> The first item is to continue to do voluntary testing, and (mandatory) testing of some populations like the military, the blood donors and so forth.
>
> The efficiency of such a program as measured by the positive predictive value is very poor. It should at least be followed by tracing contacts. I think **not** tracing contacts is unethical.
>
> What must be done in addition is to anonymously test a representative sample of the United States population in order to estimate the real magnitude of the infection, to identify high-risk groups and then concentrate on those risk groups. And then it should be decided whether to test them in a voluntary fashion, or in a mandatory routine fashion, which will be more efficient, because at least after a representative sample is tested, we should be informed.
>
> As health workers, we have a responsibility to protect the public health and use all methods to prevent the spread of AIDS using education, screening, and contact tracing. Legislation should aim to protect privacy and confidentiality by establishing criminal liabilities for negligence or intentional disclosure of test results.
>
> We must, as citizens, be concerned with human rights, but let us also remember, as an American judge once said: "My freedom to swing my arm ends where your nose begins." I suggest that by being overly careful about human rights we are forgetting our main objective, and that is to protect human lives.

In Naggan's opinion the moral obligation to prevent harm to the public (beneficence) overrides the moral obligation to respect the right to selfdetermination (autonomy).

But this does not solve the ethical conflict involved in mandatory screening for HIV. The principles of non-maleficence and justice must also be considered. Naggan does not mention justice, but he takes account of the requirement not to harm those who are tested: "legislation should aim to protect privacy and confidentiality by establishing criminal liabilities for negligence or intentional disclosure of test results".

This last requirement makes the ethical conflict complicated. Does the obligation to be beneficient, in Naggan's opinion, always override the obligation to respect autonomy, or is the relation between these two obligations dependent upon how the principle of non-maleficence is handled? Naggan is not explicit on this point, but the following interpretation, suggested by Westrin (personal communication) seems reasonable. Health care professionals either do not or do harm to those tested. (This is not quite true. The question is not one of either/or, but of degrees. Those who are tested could be more or less harmed. This complication is ignored for the moment.)

In the first case, that is, if health care professionals **do fulfill** the obligation not to harm those tested, then the obligation to respect their autonomy is overridden by the obligation to prevent harm to the general public (Fig. 3).

Groups of persons involved	Ethical principles			
	Autonomy	Non-male-ficence	Bene-ficence	Justice
Health care professionals; doctors, nurses, etc	2	Satisfied	1	[O]
Persons worth testing who do consent	[R]	R	R [O]	[R]
Persons worth testing who do not consent	R	R	R [O]	[R]
Other people being affected by the epidemic			R	[R]

Figure 3. If the principle of non-maleficence is satisfied by the health care professionals, then their obligation to respect the right to beneficence of the general public overrides their obligation to respect the right to autonomy of those who do not consent.

Groups of persons involved	Ethical principles			
	Autonomy	Non-maleficence	Beneficence	Justice
Health care professionals; doctors, nurses, etc	1	Not satisfied	2	[O]
Persons worth testing who do consent	[R]	R	R [O]	[R]
Persons worth testing who do not consent	R	R	R [O]	[R]
Other people being affected by the epidemic			R	[R]

Figure 4. If the principle of non-maleficence is not satisfied by the health care professionals, then their obligation to respect the right to autonomy of those who do not consent overrides their obligation to respect the right to beneficence of the general public.

In the second case, that is, if health care professionals **do not fulfill** the obligation of non-maleficence, i.e. they harm those tested, then the obligation to respect autonomy overrides the obligation to prevent harm to the general public (Fig. 4).

The critical factor in solving the ethical conflict raised by mandatory screening for HIV is how the testing is performed. Are those tested taken care of (with substantial pre-test and post-test counseling) and protected (by anonymous testing or with sufficient confidentiality)?

Concluding remarks

In this essay I have presented and applied a simple model designed to identify and analyze ethical conflicts. Used as an heuristic device the model provides understanding of such conflicts by identifying the persons involved, the relevant ethical principles, the implied moral obligations and moral right, and how these obligations and rights give rise to conflicts.

Sometimes this understanding goes far enough to solve the conflicts and sometimes it shows why unequivocal ethical solutions are not forthcoming. But in most cases, and this is the main value of the model, this understanding helps to overcome the paralyzing feeling of facing an unresolvable dilemma - an incentive to reexamine the situation, the alternatives and their probable consequences.

References

1. Naggan, L.: Volunteers and informed consent. Protection of the public's health and the individual's privacy rights - An unresolved conflict? The case of screening for AIDS. In: Leiter E, ed. Proceedings of the Second International Congress on Ethics in Medicine, June, 1987. New York: Beth Israel Medical Center, 1988:161-169.

2. Sinnott-Armstrong, W.: Moral dilemmas. Oxford & New York: Basil Blackwell, 1988.

3. Hermerén, G.: Kunskapens pris. Forskningsetiska problem och principer i humaniora och samhällsvetenskap. Stockholm: Forskningsrådens förlagstjänst, 1986.

4. Francoeur, R.T.: Biomedical ethics. A guide to decision making. New York: John Wiley & Sons, 1983.

5. Beauchamp, T.L., Childress, J.F.: Principles of biomedical ethics (2nd ed). New York, Oxford: Oxford University Press, 1983.

6. Gillon, R.: Philosophical medical ethics (2nd ed). Chichester: John Wiley & Sons, 1986.

7. The Appleton Consensus: Suggested International Guidelines for Decisions to Forgo Medical Treatment, 1988. (Quoted from Ugeskrift for laeger. 1989;11:669-706)

8. Fletcher, J.: Situation Ethics: The New Morality. Philadelphia: Westminster Press, 1966.

9. Russell, B.: What I believe. 1925 (Quoted from Edwards P, ed. Why I am not a Christian. London: Unwin paperbacks, 1979:43-69)

Subject Index

A

Adams-Stokes' syndrome, 69
Africa, 9,36,77
Age
   over-90, increase in surgery for, 56,81
   and rationing/limit-setting, 56–60, 80–84
AIDS. *See* HIV/AIDS, ethical issues
Alexander, 85–86
Alzheimer's disease, advances, 85
American College of Cardiology, 72
American Medical Association, 146
Amulets, folk medicine, 44
Angina pectoris, 73
Anthropology. *See* Integrity and autonomy, anthropological view
Aplastic anemia, 65,66
Arrhythmias, heart, 69–72
Asia, 79
Association of Psychiatrists, 194
Atomism, 9,14
   vs. holism, and guidelines/codes of ethics, 140
Autonomy, 1,3–9,13–15,19,47–51
   vs. benificence, 3,9,18
   children, 50
   clinical freedom, doctor's, 103–104,109,111
   as concept and principle, 4
   constraints to, 5
   deficiencies as moral guide, 8–9
   privatism, atomism, 9,14
   doctor–patient relationship, 115, 116
   of embryo, 50–51
   and epidemiology, 174
   vs. integrity, 15–16
   legal basis for, 6–9
   limitations on patient's claims to, 13–15
   community, 14–15
   medical ethics and ordinary morality, 24,27–29
   community, 29–30
   patient
     and integrity, 10–13,16,17–18
     treatment withdrawal, 92
   philosophical roots, 7–8
   physicians', 13
   as self-rule, 4,5,48
   social and political sources, 5–6
   see also Clinical freedom, physicians'; Integrity and autonomy, anthropological view
AZT, 183

B

Battin, Margaret, 80
Being vs. doing, 49
Benificence vs. autonomy, 3,9,18
Bill of Rights, 6
Blood as metaphor, 37–38
Body–self, notion of, 35–40
Bone marrow transplantation, treatment priorities, 65–68
   allogeneic, HLA-matched, 65–66

215

Bone marrow transplantation *(contd.)*
  aplastic anemia, 65,66
  autologous, 66-68
  complications, 68
  costs, 67
  leukemia, 65-68
  treatment processing and conditioning, 65-66
Bororo (Africa), integrity and autonomy, 36
Buddhist integration of Western medicine, 43
Bypass surgery, 73

C
Callahan, Dan, 80-83,85,86
Canada
  Greek immigrants, Montreal, 143
  Medical Research Council, 129
Categorical cutoffs in medical care, 82
Categorical imperative, 29
Children
  AIDS, ethical issues, 184,185
  autonomy, 50
China, 118,120
  Cultural Revolution, 118
Chronic care, rationing, 84-85
Clinical freedom, physicians', 89-100,103-112
  application to clinical situations, 105-111
    in daily work, 106-107
    marginal situations, 107,108
    psychotic patients, 111
    research involving patients, 107-109,110
  autonomy, 103-104,109,111
  economy and resource aspects, 105
  ethical considerations, 90-96
  legal considerations, 90-96,105
  limit-setting and cost-containment, 90,96-98
  medical audit for improving standards, 98-100
  paternalism, 112
  U.K., 96
    HMOs, 97-98
    NHS, 89,96
  U.S., 90,96-98
    peer review organizations, 100
Code of conduct, epidemiology, 126-127,132-133,175-176; *see also* Guidelines/codes of ethics, multi-cultural view
Communication in health-care encounters, 41-45
Community and autonomy, 14-15, 29-30
Computerized data, researcher access to, and informed consent, 160
Condorcet, 56
Confidentiality. *See* Privacy/confidentiality
Conflicts of interest in epidemiology, 168-169
Consent, informed, 50
Consequentialist ethics, 25-27
Constitution, U.S., 6
Corporate control of data, work-related illnesses, 129-130
Cost(s)
  bone marrow transplantation, treatment priorities, 67
  limit-setting in medical care, 56
Cost-benefit analysis
  heart disorders, priorities in advanced technology, 74
  rationing and priority setting in medical care, 81-82,84
Cost-containment and clinical freedom, physicians', 90,96-98
Crick, Francis, 85

Cultural setting, medical ethics and ordinary morality, 24
  relativism, 30
Culture, anthropological sense, 34–35
  and integrity, 40–41
  see also Guidelines/codes of ethics, multi-cultural view
Cuna Indians (Panama), 37

D

Data, raw and analyzed, control/ownership, 129–130
Data, researcher access to, and informed consent, 1,153,159–164
  computerized data, 160
  hepatitis B antigen study, retrospective interest in sexual practices, 161
  privacy, infringement of, 160
  prospective clinical studies, 159
  retrospective studies and, 160–162
Death certificate, AIDS, ethical issues, 199–200
Decision-making, categorical vs. individual, limit-setting in medical care, 61–64
Declaration of Geneva, 190,196
Defensive medicine (U.S.), 94
Defibrillating pacemakers, 71
Deficiencies as moral guide, autonomy, 8–9
Dentist, AIDS risk to, 200
Deontology, 25,27
Developing countries. *See* Third World
Dignity, doctor–patient relationship, 120–121
Disease as disintegration, 10–12
Doctor–patient relationship, 12, 115–121
  autonomy, 115,116

China, 118,120
  Cultural Revolution, 118
  contract vs. covenant, 9
  dignity, 120–121
  epidemiology, ethical aspects, 152
  Jewish (Talmudic) law, 117–120, 121
  paternalism, 115–117
  see also Clinical freedom, physicians'
DRGs, 96–98
Drug abuse, parenteral, AIDS, ethical issues, 179–186,193
Drug trials, placebo-controlled, AIDS, ethical issues, 200,201

E

ECG, invention, 69
Ecology, anthropological sense, 34, 35
Economic vs. moral solutions, limit-setting in medical care, 57
Elderly. *See* Age
Embryo
  autonomy, 50–51
  integrity, 50–51
Epidemic diseases, 126
Epidemiology, ethical issues, 123–134,151–157,167–177
  autonomy, conflict with, 174
  code of conduct, need for, 132–133
  conflicts of interest between parties, 168–169
  data, raw and analyzed, control/ownership, 129–130
  doctor–patient relationship, 152
  epidemic disease, 126
  ethics guidelines/codes, 126–127, 131–132,175–176
  informed consent, 169–172

Epidemiology *(contd.)*
  intervention, responsibility for, 155-156
    plasma storage, 155-156
  methodological issues, 168-169
  number of subjects, 152-154
  observational research, 154-155
    vs. experimental, 152,154
  politicians, responsibility, 173-174
  presentation of results, 130-131
    least publishable units, 131
  privacy and confidentiality, 128-129
    death certificates, 128
  public health, 152
  researchers, responsibility, 173-174
  responsibilities to research subjects, 127-128
    review committees, 127
  social philosophy, 174-175
  status of, 172-173
    Third World, 172
    USSR, 172
  surveillance vs. research, 125
  Sweden, 131,151-153,174
    twin study of mental health problems, 123
  Third World health problems, 134
  U.K., 132
Ethical contract theories, 27
Europe, AIDS, ethical issues, 183
Euthanasia
  animals vs. humans, 167-168
  Nazi Germany, 85-86

F
Family planning, 141-142
Folk medicine, 38
  amulets, 44
Foucault, Michel, 141

Freedom. *See* Clinical freedom, physicians'
Fuchs, Victor, 78

G
Geertz, Clifford, 36
Germany, Nazi
  atrocities, 154
  euthanasia program, 85-86
Gillon, Raanan, 80
Ginzberg, Eli, 97
Gordon, D.R., 141
Guidelines/codes of ethics, epidemiology, 126-127,132-133, 175-176
Guidelines/codes of ethics, multicultural view, 137-148
  adaptability, 139,140
  compromise, 139
  family planning, 141-142
  general to specific guidelines necessary, 144
  Japan, 142
  nonmedical issues, 147
  pesticides in developing countries, 146-147
  public health and confidentiality, 144-145
  purpose, 145-146
  right-based bioethics, 143-144
  social/political issues, micro vs. macro, 146-147
  universality, 145,146
  Western domination and need for cultural sensitivity, 138-140,143,147
    atomism vs. holism, 140
    emphasis on contract, 142
    individualist emphasis, 140-144
    paternalism, 142

H
Health maintenance organizations, U.K., 97-98

SUBJECT INDEX

Heart disease, mortality, 69
Heart disorders, priorities in advanced technology, 69–75
   angina pectoris and diabetes, 73
   bypass surgery, 73
   risk factor patients, 73
   arrhythmias, 69–72
   cost–benefit/cost–efficiency analyses, 74
   invasive procedures, 72
   HIV-positive patient, 72
   pacemakers, no reuse in U.S., 70
   unrealiability of equipment, 71
Heinz, John III (Senator), 98
Helsinki Declaration, 127,154,169, 170
   World Medical Association, 30
Hepatitis B antigen study, retrospective interest in sexual practices, 161
Hippocrates, 145
HIV/AIDS, ethical issues, 1,13,72, 126,145,146,155,179–180
   clinical practice, 199–201
   confidentiality, 185–186
   death certificate, 199–200
   dentist, risk to, 200
   drug abuse, parenteral, 179–186, 193
     needle exchange programs, 180,193–195
     treatment as AIDS prevention, 183–184,195
   drug trials, placebo-controlled, 200,201
   ethical conflicts, 180,189
   informing sexual partners, 199
   medical profession and, 179–180,189,190–192,195–196
     Sweden, 191–192
   needle-stick, medical personnel, 200
   patient integrity, 180
   political aspects, 179–180,189, 191,192–193,197
   need for guidelines, 197
   Sweden, 192–193
   public health measures, 203–213
     high-risk group identification, U.S., 210
     model for identification and analysis of ethical conflicts, 205–206
     prevention of transmission, 205
     surveillance, 203
     testing, mandatory vs. voluntary, 203–204,207–210
   research area, 184–185
   steady-state equilibrium, establishment at, 201
   surgeon, refusal to operate, 200
   surveillance, 203
   testing
     compulsory, and green card system, 180,201
     refusal, 199
   therapeutic agents, 184
   transfusion recipient, 200
HMOs, U.K., 97–98
Homosexual men, AIDS, 183

I

Illich, Ivan, 73
Individual cure, limit-setting in medical care, 58,60–61
Individualist emphasis
   guidelines/codes of ethics, multi-cultural view, 140–144
   and rationing of medical care, 83–85
Individual vs. society, anthropological point of view, 35–40
Industrial Epidemiology Forum, 131–132,138,140
Information, ownership/control of, 129–130; *see also* Data, researcher access to, and informed consent

Informed consent, 50
  epidemiology, ethical aspects, 169–172
    feedback, 171
  medical ethics and ordinary morality, 24,27–29
  see also Data, researcher access to, and informed consent
Institutional Review Boards, Israel, 163,164
Integrity, 1,3,8,10–13,15–18,47–51
  vs. autonomy, 15–16
  being vs. doing, 49
  disease as disintegration, 10–12
  embryo, 50–51
  etymology, 10,47
  medical ethics and ordinary mortality, 24,27–29
  of patient as person, 10–13,16
    and AIDS, 180
  physical, 11
  physician, 10,12–13,16–18
    fidelity, 18
    patient autonomy, 17–18
  psychological, 11
  violation or loss of, 49
Integrity and autonomy, anthropological view, 33
  body–self, notion of, 35–40
  communication in health-care encounters, 41–45
  cultures, clash of, 40–41
  individual vs. society, 35–40
    non-Western cultures, 36–37, 39,40
    Western cultures, 36–40
Intensive care unit admission criteria, 62
International Epidemiological Association, 124,126–127,132
Inuits, 143
Invasive procedures, heart disorders, 72
  HIV-positive patient, 72
Iron lung, 90

Israel
  Institutional Review Boards, 163,164
  Law for Protection of Privacy, 163
  retrospective study of polymyositis-dermatomyositis, 160
  Supreme Court, 118

J
Japan
  guidelines/codes of ethics, multi-cultural view, 142
  integrity and autonomy, anthropological point of view, 36
Jehovah's Witnesses, 44
Jewish law and doctor–patient relationship, 117–120,121

K
Kant, Immanuel, 7,25,26
  categorical imperative, 29
Karolinska Institute, 152
Kirmeyer, L.J., 141,142

L
Legal considerations
  autonomy, 6–9
  clinical freedom, physicians', 90–96,105
Leprosy, 126
Leukemia, bone marrow transplantation, treatment priorities, 65–68
Lifeboat ethics, 26
Limit-setting in medical care, 55–64
  aging/the elderly, 56–60
  and clinical freedom, physicians', 90,96–98
    rationing, 97
  costs, 56

decision-making, categorical vs. individual, 61-64
economic vs. moral solutions, 57
individual cure, 58,60-61
progress, definition of, 56
quality-of-life considerations, 61
Litigation and treatment withdrawal, 94
Living wills, 91
Locke, John, 7

M
Maimonides, 117,119,145
Mammographic screening, 156
Marcel, Gabriel, 10
Massachusetts Supreme Court, 93
Mayans, Mexico, 37
Mayo Clinic, 56,81
Medical directive, proposed, 9
Medical ethics and ordinary morality, 23-25,30
  autonomy, 24,27-29
    community, 29-30
  cultural relativism, 30
  cultural setting, 24
  ethical contract theories, 27
  human right to change one's mind, 24
  informed consent, 24,27-29
  integrity, 24,27-29
  management of biomedical ethics decisions, 27-28
  theoretical ethics, 25-26
Medicine
  Buddhist integration of Western medicine, 43
  as cultural product, 35
  folk, 38,44
  non-Western culture, 36-37,39
Men, homosexual, AIDS, ethical issues, 183
Mental health problems, Swedish twin study, 123

Menzel, Paul, 81
Mexico, 37
Military expenditures vs. rationing and priority setting in medical care, 77
Mill, John Stuart, 7
Mortality, heart disease, 69

N
Naggan, Lechaim, 203-205
Nazi Germany
  atrocities, 154
  euthanasia program, 85-86
Needle exchange programs and AIDS, 180,193-195
  WHO, 194
Needle-stick, medical personnel, AIDS ethical issues, 200
Negative rights, 7
Neisser, 95
Netherlands, 91
New Guinea, 36
New Jersey
  AIDS, 183
  Supreme Court, 93
New York City, AIDS, 182-183
New York State Division of Substance Abuse Services, 182

O
Oath of Hippocrates, 190
Observational research, epidemiology, ethical aspects, 154-155
  vs. experimental, 152,154
Ordinary morality. *See* Medical ethics and ordinary morality

P
Pacemakers, cardiac
  defibrillating, 71
  reuse, 70

Pacemakers, cardiac *(contd.)*
   Sweden, 69–71
Panama, 37
Paternalism
   clinical freedom, physicians', 112
   doctor–patient relationship, 115–117
   guidelines/codes of ethics, multi-cultural view, 142
Peer review organizations, 100
Percival, 145
Pesticides in developing countries, 146–147
Philosophical roots, autonomy, 7–8
Physical integrity, 11
Physician
   autonomy, 13
   integrity, 10,12–13,16–18
   see also Clinical freedom, physicians'; Doctor–patient relationship
Plasma storage, 155–156
Poliomyelitis, 90
Political aspects, AIDS, 179–180, 189,191,192–193,197
Politicians, epidemiology, ethical aspects, 173–174
Polymyositis-dermatomyositis, retrospective study, Israel, 160
Polyneuritis, 90
Premature newborns, minimum weight limits for aggressive treatment, 62
Priority setting in medical care, 53–54
   informing patients and public, 54
   see also Bone marrow transplantation, treatment priorities; Heart disorders, priorities in advanced technology; Rationing and priority setting in medical care

Privacy/confidentiality
   AIDS, 185–186
   epidemiology, 128–129
      death certificates, 128
   and informed consent, 160
   and public health, 144–145
Privatism and autonomy, 9,14
Progress, definition of, and limit-setting in medical care, 56
Prospective clinical studies, researcher access to data and informed consent, 159
Psychological integrity, 11
Psychotic patients, clinical freedom, physicians', 111
Publication, medical research, 131
Public health
   AIDS, ethical issues, 203–213
   and confidentiality, guidelines/codes of ethics, 144–145
   epidemiology, ethical aspects, 152

Q
Quality-of-life considerations and limit-setting in medical care, 61
Quarantine, 126
Quinlan, Karen, 93

R
Rand Corp., 203
Rationing and priority setting in medical care, 77–86
   age cutoff, 80–84
   categorical cutoffs, 82
   chronic care, 84–85
   and clinical freedom, physicians', 97
   cost–benefit analysis, 81–82,84
   disparities within Western countries, 79
   global context, 77

vs. military expenditures, 77
patient individuality in Western
medical tradition, 83–85
U.S., 85,86
Western vs. underdeveloped
countries, 77,79
Researchers' responsibility, epidemiology, 173–174
Retrospective studies
of polymyositis-dermatomyositis, Israel, 160
researcher access to data and informed consent, 160–162
Rights-based bioethics, guidelines/codes of ethics, multi-cultural view, 143–144
Rights, negative, 7
Right-to-know legislation, U.S., 130
Royal College of Physicians (U.K.), 99
Royal College of Surgeons (U.K.), 100

S

Saikewicz case, 93
"Salami" publishing, 131
Screening, mammographic, 156
Self-consciousness, 36
Shaw, G.B., 120
Social philosophy, epidemiology, ethical aspects, 174–175
Society for Epidemiological Research, 127,131,132
Sri Lanka, 43
Suicide, legalization, 81
Sumner, 27
Surgeon, refusal to operate, and AIDS, 200
Surveillance
AIDS, ethical issues, 203
vs. research, epidemiology, ethical issues, 125
Sweden, 44,45,50,62

AIDS, ethical issues
medical profession, 191–192
politics, 192–193
Board of Malpractice, 195
epidemiology, ethical aspects, 131,151–153,174
Medical Ethics Committee, 194
Minister of Health and Social Welfare, 193
National Board of Health and Welfare, 70,191
National Medical Ethics Council, 51
pacemakers, cardiac, 69–71
Physicians against AIDS, 191, 194
Turkish women in, 41,43,44
twin study of mental health problems, ethical issues, 123
Swedish Medical Association, 180, 194
Swedish Society of Medicine, 194
Syphilis, 19th century research, 95

T

Talmudic law and doctor–patient relationship, 117–120,121
Technology, advanced. *See* Heart disorders, priorities in advanced technology
Theoretical ethics, 25–26
Third World
epidemiology, ethical aspects, 134,172
pesticides, 146–147
Transfusion recipient, AIDS ethical issues, 200
Transplantation, donor, 1; *see also* Bone marrow transplantation, treatment priorities
Treatment withdrawal, 90–94
as medical decision, 91
patient autonomy, 92

Treatment withdrawal *(contd.)*
  U.K., 91–94
  U.S., 91–93
    litigation, 94
Turkish women in Sweden, 41,43, 44
Twin studies, mental health problems, 123

U
U.K., 85
  clinical freedom, physicians', 96
  HMOs, 97–98
  NHS, 89,96
  epidemiology, ethical issues, 132
  General Medical Council, 99
  Royal College of Physicians of London, 99
  Royal College of Surgeons, 100
  treatment withdrawal, 91–94
U.N., 146,175
U.S., 59,62
  clinical freedom, physicians', 90, 96–98
  defensive medicine, 94
  Industrial Epidemiology Forum, 131–132
  National Commission for the Protection of Human Subjects of Biomedical and Behavioral Research, 162
  percentage of GNP devoted to medical care, 56
  desperately ill, 60
  Public Health Service, 203
  rationing and priority setting in medical care, 85,86
  right-to-know legislation, 130
  treatment withdrawal, 91–93
  waste in medical expenditure, 57
U.S.S.R., epidemiology, ethical aspects, 172
Utilitarianism, 25–27,45

W
Wallace, William, 95
Waste in medical expenditure, U.S., 57
Western cultures
  integrity and autonomy, anthropological point of view, 36–40
  need for cultural sensitivity, guidelines/codes of ethics, 138–140,143,147
  vs. underdeveloped countries, priority setting in medical care, 77,79
"Wholistic" physician–patient relationship, 12
Wills, living, 91
Wojtyla, Karol, 10
Work-related illnesses, corporate control of data, 129–130
World Health Organization, 146, 175,190
  AIDS, ethical issues, 181
  needle exchange programs, 194
World Medical Association, 30